AF582592

Global Mental Health: Equity Now

Mariyak

Copyright © 2024 by Mariyak

All rights reserved. No part of this book may be reproduced in any manner whatso-ever without written permission except in the case of brief quotations embodied in critical articles and reviews.

First Printing, 2024

Table of Contents

Chapter one: Background

1.1. Introduction

Mental and substance use disorders are a global public health problem. They are one of the leading causes of disability adjusted life years (DALYs) worldwide (Whiteford et al., 2013). The global burden of mental illness accounts for 32·4% of years lived with disability (YLDs) and 13·0% of DALYs (Vigo, Thornicroft, & Atun, 2016). For all mental disorders, depression takes the leading share (Whiteford et al., 2013). Depression is also common during the perinatal period and deserves special attention. In addition to the suffering, severe distress and significant impairment it causes the affected women, it can also have a negative impact on obstetric and child outcomes (Grigoriadis et al., 2013; Hanlon et al., 2009; Patel & Prince, 2006; Rahman, Bunn, Lovel, & Creed, 2007; Stein et al., 2014).

The gap between treatment need and the allocation of human resources for mental health problems in low and middle income countries (LMICs) is large (Kohn, Saxena, Levav, & Saraceno, 2004). Because of a shortage of mental health professionals and other reasons, only a fraction of those affected by mental disorders receive appropriate treatment (WHO, 2011). A study from Ethiopia showed that, of those with severe mental illness, only 10% have ever received modern treatment for their mental health problem (Alem et al., 2009). For depression the treatment gap is expected to be even higher since it is less likely to cause disruptive behavior, which is one of the main reasons for presentation to a mental health clinic. A finding from a study on postnatal women in southern Ethiopia showed that only 4.2% of women with high level of depressive symptoms had obtained mental health care indicating that the treatment gap for maternal common mental disorders is high (Azale, Fekadu, & Hanlon, 2016).

The World Health Organisation (WHO) launched the mental health Gap Action Programme (mhGAP) to reduce the mental health treatment gap in LMICs (WHO, 2008). Ethiopia was one of the countries to pilot the program. Working with the district health office and local stakeholders, the Programme for improving mental health care (PRIME) in Ethiopia (Lund et al., 2012) trained all primary health care workers in the Sodo district, southern Ethiopia, on the mhGAP base course. Since 2014, primary health care (PHC) workers in the district have been treating people with priority mental disorders - psychosis, depressive disorders, alcohol use disorder, suicidality and epilepsy (Fekadu et al., 2016)- using the mhGAP Intervention Guide (mhGAP-IG) (WHO, 2010; WHO 2016). Training of PHC workers on WHO's mhGAP has been very successful in decreasing the treatment gap for severe mental illness in the district (Hailemariam, Fekadu, Medhin, Prince, & Hanlon, 2019; Hanlon et al., 2020) but less successful for internalizing disorders like depression (Fekadu et al., 2017; Rathod et al., 2018).

The mhGAP-IG, which is evidence based intervention guide developed by the WHO to assist in implementation of mhGAP (WHO, 2016), has a different approach when it comes to management of pregnant and breastfeeding women. For pregnant and breastfeeding women, if depression is identified by PHC clinicians, it recommends psychosocial support as the first line management. The motivation for this advice is to protect the foetus/baby from unnecessary exposure to psychotropic medications, but might make providing care difficult for the PHC workers who are used to bio-medical model of medicine. If psychosocial support is not successful in improving symptoms then PHC workers can prescribe antidepressants at the lowest effective dose (mhGAP-IG, WHO, 2016).

Detection of depression in PHC is very low (Fekadu et al., 2017; Rathod et al., 2018). The same is likely to be true for perinatal depression, including antenatal depression. An unpublished report from a study done in southern part of Ethiopia shows that the prevalence of clinical depression (i.e. Major Depressive Disorder (MDD)) in antenatal care (ANC) clinics is 3.9% (Girma, 2013), but our participant recruitment experience in the initial iteration of the current study shows that the rate of detection is very much lower than that, if not nil. This required the current study objective to be revised. Thus this research aims to gather evidence on the current practice of detection of pregnant women with moderate-severe depression in the Sodo district and to explore potential solutions to the identified challenges.

1.2. Research questions

1. What are the challenges in detection of moderate to severe depression in pregnant women in PHC settings in the Sodo district, rural Ethiopia, where mhGAP is being implemented?
2. How could the PHC based detection of moderate to severe depression be improved to meet the needs of the pregnant women?

1.3. Aim

The aim of this study is to understand the entry into pathways of care for pregnant women with moderate to severe depression to receive mhGAP-based care in the Sodo district, rural Ethiopia, and to identify potential solutions for improving detection of cases.

1.4. Specific objectives

1. To assess challenges, from the perspectives of pregnant women and PHC workers, in detection of moderate to severe depression in pregnant women in PHC settings where mhGAP is being implemented.
2. To explore PHC workers perspective on possible approaches to solving the identified problems.

Chapter two: Literature review

2.1. Epidemiology of antenatal depression

2.1.1. Prevalence

Major Depressive Disorder (MDD) is a leading cause of disease burden for women of childbearing age, but the burden of MDD attributable to perinatal depression is not yet known (Woody, Ferrari, Siskind, Whiteford, & Harris, 2017). It is difficult to estimate the exact prevalence as studies are not uniform in their usage of the term depression. Some studies use the term depression to refer to high burden of depressive symptoms endorsed on a depression screening instrument, which may or may not be equivalent to a diagnosis of MDD, while others refer to clinically significant depression or diagnosis of MDD. The prevalence estimates from studies which used depression screening instruments are significantly higher than prevalence estimates which used diagnostic instruments (Girma, 2013; Ayano, Tesfaw, & Shumet, 2019; Woody et al., 2017).

The prevalence of perinatal depression is significantly higher in women from low and middle income countries (LMICs) than from high income countries (HICs) (Woody et al., 2017). A systematic review showed that the overall pooled prevalence of perinatal depression is 11.9% globally (Woody et al., 2017). This figure is much lower than the prevalence estimates from LMICs which indicate that the prevalence of antenatal depression ranges from 15.6% - 25.8%, and estimate the prevalence of postnatal depression to be above 19.5% (Fisher et al., 2012; Gelaye, Rondon, Araya, & Williams, 2016).

Systematic reviews also show similar findings from Ethiopia. The pooled prevalence of perinatal depression is around 25.8% (Mersha, Abebe, Sori, & Abegaz, 2018). When considering antenatal depression separately, it ranged from 21 – 24% (Ayano et al., 2019; Zegeye et al., 2018). The prevalence is higher in studies conducted using depression screening instruments in clinical settings (25.8%) than community settings (15.5%)(Ayano et al., 2019). In a study from rural Ethiopia, the prevalence of clinical depression (MDD) made by psychiatric nurses during pregnancy was 3.9% in PHC settings (Girma, 2013).

2.1.2. Risk factors

From systematic reviews (Fisher et al., 2012; Gelaye et al., 2016), identified risk factors for perinatal common mental disorders in LMICs are childhood abuse, socioeconomic disadvantage, maternal low educational attainment, unplanned pregnancy, being younger, being unmarried, lacking intimate partner empathy and support, having hostile in-laws, experiencing intimate partner violence (IPV), having insufficient emotional and practical support and having a history of mental health problems. In some settings, giving birth to a girl baby (Patel, Rodrigues, & DeSouza, 2002) is considered a risk factor. Protective factors identified in the same study were: having more education, having a permanent job, being of the ethnic majority and having a kind, trustworthy intimate partner (Fisher et al., 2012).

Similarly in Ethiopia, a previous history of depression, poor socioeconomic status, lack of social support, being unmarried, obstetric complications in previous and/or current pregnancy, an unplanned pregnancy and experiencing marital conflict and IPV were the major factors associated with perinatal depression (Ayano et al., 2019; Mersha et al., 2018; Zegeye et al., 2018).

2.1.3. Impact

There is emerging evidence that stress, anxiety, or depression during pregnancy can alter the development of a woman's fetus and her child, with an increased risk for subsequent child emotional and behavioral problems (Glover, O'Donnell, O'Connor, & Fisher, 2018). Available studies from LMICs indicate that perinatal depression has significant clinical and developmental consequences for children (Gelaye et al., 2016). A consistent finding in most studies is that antenatal depression is associated with low birth weight and preterm delivery (Gelaye et al., 2016). An Ethiopian study showed a relationship between antenatal common mental disorders and prolonged labor of more than 24 hours and delayed initiation of breastfeeding (Hanlon et al., 2009). Perinatal depression is also associated with childhood stunting and underweight, stopping breastfeeding early, insecure infant-mother attachment and increased diarrheal episodes and other childhood illnesses (Gelaye et al., 2016). There is also some evidence on its relationship to childhood obesity (McConley et al., 2011) and neurodevelopmental outcomes (Stein et al., 2014) but these effects are not well studied in LMICs.

2.1.4. Detection

Detection of depression in PHC in LMICs is very low (Fekadu et al., 2017; Rathod et al., 2018). A study from Ethiopia, which used a depression symptom rating scale (patient health questionnaire - 9 item version (PHQ-9) (Kroenke & Spitzer, 2002)), showed that over 98% of cases with probable PHQ-9 depression were undetected in rural PHC settings (Fekadu et al., 2017). There is little reason to expect the situation to be any different for perinatal depression, including antenatal depression. An unpublished report from a study done in the same region shows that the prevalence of clinical depression (i.e. Major Depressive Disorder (MDD)) in antenatal care (ANC) clinics is 3.9% (Girma, 2013), but our participant recruitment experience in an earlier iteration of the current study shows that the rate of detection is very much lower than that if not nil.

2.2 Barriers to detecting depression in primary care

Recognition of depression in primary health care (PHC), where time and resources are limited, is challenging. Detection remained low even after a trial of integration of mental health care into primary care, following training of PHC workers on WHO's mhGAP-IG (Jordans & Luitel, 2019; Rathod et al., 2018). Emotional responses to suffering vary from place to place and that, coupled with lack of acceptance of depression as a disorder, both by medical professionals and the wider community, makes depression difficult to identify and measure globally (Williams, Sarker, & Ferdous, 2018). The under-recognition of depression contributes to the huge treatment gap, as only a fraction of those affected by depression receive appropriate treatment (Thornicroft et al., 2017). The barriers to depression care can be roughly categorized into four levels: client level barriers, provider level barriers, system level barriers (Byatt et al., 2013; Byatt et al., 2012; Hirschfeld et al., 1997; Mitchell, 2010) and illness level influences (Mitchell, 2010).

2.2.1. Client level barriers

Recognition of depression, or any distress for that matter, depends in part on the reporting of symptoms during a consultation. A major client factor that appears to influence detection is how the person with depression experiences and describes his or her symptoms (Mitchell, 2010). This is especially true for detection of mild to moderate depression, which is more common in PHC settings, where observable signs might be absent. It is equally important that disclosure of psychological symptoms happen early in the consultation as depressed patients who mention depressive symptoms early in the consultation are much more likely to be diagnosed as having depression (Tylee, Freeling, Kerry, & Burns, 1995). This might be because for those who mention psychological symptoms early in consultation, their psychological symptoms are their presenting complaints and they are less likely to have comorbid physical illness which may mask the diagnosis of depression (Floyd, 1997). The prevalence of MDD in PHC in southern Ethiopia was 5.9%, according to the gold standard psychiatric nurse assessment (Hanlon et al., 2015). However, patients around the world usually do not complain of depression in PHC settings (Cornford, Hill, & Reilly, 2007; Yeung, Chang, Gresham Jr, Nierenberg, & Fava, 2004). To support this, data from ten European countries showed low rates of spontaneous emotional complaints from patients in a primary care setting (Verhaak & Bensing, 2007). Nonetheless, most patients will discuss psychological symptoms if asked (Simon, VonKorff, Piccinelli, Fullerton, & Ormel, 1999; Williams Jr et al., 1999).

Patients' views about their depressive symptoms may be different from conventional medical views (Cornford et al., 2007; Yeung et al., 2004). As an example, in a qualitative community study done in Ethiopia (Hanlon, Whitley, Wondimagegn, Alem, & Prince, 2010), the distress in a pregnant woman was attributed to the vulnerability of the pregnant woman to physical and supernatural misfortune, in addition to socioeconomic and health burdens of pregnancy. In that study, only few women talked about levels of distress that were considered to be abnormal and needing a specialized intervention, i.e. modern treatment (Hanlon et al., 2010).

Patients may be reluctant to seek help and disclose symptoms due to various reasons. Some of them are: belief that the PHC worker is not the right person to talk to or mental health symptoms should not be discussed at all (Mitchell, 2010), feeling that there is little the PHC worker could do, feeling of being able to cope without emotional help, psychological embarrassment and hesitation to trouble the PHC worker (Cape & McCulloch, 1999). Most of the time depression presents with somatic symptoms rather than/in addition to psychological complaints and patients tend to disclose somatic complaints only. This results in under-recognition of depression in PHC (Tylee et al., 1995). A WHO primary care study concluded that "it seems that many patients assume that a physical symptom is almost a requirement in order to be seen at a health facility" (Patel, 1996), and this might lead to a tendency to express distress with physical symptoms. Lower educational levels of patients create a knowledge barrier which results in low awareness of emotional symptoms leading to a failure to recognize the symptoms and under-estimating the severity of depression (Hirschfeld et al., 1997). Some do not want to disclose symptoms because of fear of stigma associated with the label of mental illness (Hirschfeld et al., 1997). Patients want to protect their privacy and personal integrity and this also impedes the diagnostic process (Pollock, 2007). In a study from Nepal, some of the most frequently reported barriers for depression care, which can be linked to low detection were: concern that one might be seen as 'crazy', dislike of talking about one's own feelings, emotions or thoughts, and concern that one might be seen as weak for having mental health problems (Luitel, 2017).There is also a similar finding from a study on postpartum women in Ethiopia (Azale, Fekadu, & Hanlon, 2016).

2.2.2. Provider level barriers

A major provider factor that influences detection is how the clinician interviews the patient (Goldberg, Jenkins, Millar, & Faragher, 1993). History taking about depression has been found to be directly associated with the likelihood of a diagnosis of depression and provision of acceptable treatment for it. Many patients have commented on suboptimal communication behaviors from clinicians (Maguire, 2002) with poor interview and diagnostic skills influencing detection (Goldberg et al., 1993). Some studies indicate that clinicians appear to miss most cues and concerns and adopt behaviors that discourage disclosure (Deveugele, Derese, & De Maeseneer, 2002; Petersen, 2000; Zimmermann, Del Piccolo, & Finset, 2007). Communication strategies that predicted successful recognition of depression are the use of broad, open ended psychosocial questions and a proportion of the interview devoted to emotional problems (Carney et al., 1999). Insufficient undergraduate and postgraduate training as well as insufficient time for consultations will influence one's ability to identify depression (Hirschfeld et al., 1997; Mitchell, 2010). According to an article from South Africa (Petersen, 2000), PHC workers lack of skill and resource to deal with emotional problems is one factor for providing largely bio-medical care in primary care settings. PHC workers who had obtained mental health training on mhGAP-IG were more likely to diagnose priority mental health conditions when compared with baseline data (Jordans & Luitel, 2019), but diagnosis of depression still remained low. It is not only skill that is important but clinician attitude also contributes as a barrier to identification of depression (Mitchell, 2010). For example, clinicians have been shown to harbour stigmatising attitudes towards people with mental illness (Kohrt et al., 2018).

It is important to remember that patient and clinician communications are related with one another (Mitchell, 2010). Patient cues are influenced by PHC worker's behavior, decreasing with increased number of medical questions and other doctor led behaviors and increasing with more patient centered behaviors, such as empathic statements or directive questioning about psychological issues (Del Piccolo, Saltini, Zimmermann, & Dunn, 2000; Goldberg et al., 1993; Ishikawa et al., 2002).

Another important predictor of detection in primary care is the amount of contact the provider has with the patient. Some studies show that cases seen five or more times during the previous year, by the same health care worker, were more likely to be correctly identified as depressed, compared with those patients not seen in the previous year. But even in the presence of frequent contact, the therapeutic relationship dictates recognition, with a poor therapeutic relationship, noted by either the patient or provider, decreasing the chance of recognition (MItchell, 2010).

The National Depressive and Manic-Depressive Association consensus statement on the under-treatment of depression, published in 1997, lists some of these additional factors as provider level barriers to the detection of depression: limited provider training in interpersonal skills, belief in the myth that psychiatric disorders are not "real" illnesses, inadequate time to evaluate and treat depression, psychiatric disorders taking more time to diagnose and treat than many other medical conditions, and a fear of offending the patient (Hirschfeld et al., 1997). Some PHC workers also argue against the medicalization of human distress or the use of antidepressants (Naqvi & Khan, 2005).

2.2.3. Illness related influences

There is some evidence that clinicians find mental illness difficult to deal with and awkward to diagnose (Mitchell, 2010). Some evidence indicates that PHC workers may be reluctant to code patients as depressed (Naqvi & Khan, 2005; Rost, Smith, Matthews, & Guise, 1994). Physical complaints thought to have a psychological basis are also perceived as difficult (Carson, Stone, Warlow, & Sharpe, 2004; Hahn, 2001).

Somatization and presenting with medically unexplained symptoms are some of the reasons for lower detection of depression in PHC (Coyne, Klinkman, Gallo, & Schwenk, 1997). A cross sectional survey in eight health centres in Ethiopia indicated that detection of depression was extremely low (< 2%) and that all cases of depression diagnosed by PHC workers during the study period presented with psychological symptoms (Fekadu et al., 2017) which indirectly suggesting that those presenting with somatic symptoms are missed.

Depression in PHC is mostly mild to moderate in severity (Schwenk, Klinkman, & Coyne, 1998), and the detection of mild disorders is a challenge because symptoms do not differ greatly from those of healthy but stressed individuals. Determining the boundary between a clinical disorder and subclinical symptoms is complex, and non-mental health specialists report difficulty distinguishing between distress caused by significant life stressors and psychiatric illness like depression (Johnston et al., 2007). Higher severity of depression is associated with greater recognition in PHC (Naqvi & Khan, 2005). A study from rural Ethiopia showed that depression cases identified by PHC clinicians were those with high symptom burden, suicidality and functional impairment (Habtamu et al., 2019).

The presence of comorbidity may decrease recognition, but there is also evidence to the contrary or that co-morbidity might even increase recognition. One hypothesis is that somatic complaints might cause clinicians to focus on physical rather than mental symptoms (Mitchell, 2010). Accumulating evidence suggests that somatic symptoms should be counted towards depression even when another physical illness is present (Stewart et al., 2009). Seaburn et al (2005) suggests that only a minority of clinicians choose to explore the issues in more detail when faced with diagnostic difficulties (Seaburn et al., 2005) which is likely to occur in patients with comorbid medical conditions or medically unexplained symptoms.

2.2.4. System level barriers

Depression is a chronic illness which is characterized by periods of remission and relapse and its care fits well in the chronic care model. It follows that health care facilities must be equipped with the necessary organizational and administrative support to provide quality chronic care.

Lack of time and high work load may be a barrier to adequate attention being given to depression in PHC. Inadequate undergraduate/postgraduate and on-the-job training may also affect the knowledge, skill and confidence of PHC workers to identify and care for patients with depression (Hirschfeld et al., 1997; Mitchell, 2010).

Effectiveness of universal screening of people for depression in primary care settings has a mixed evidence base, despite being appealing because most people with depression will present at primary care. The evidence from a meta-analysis indicates that, without organizational enhancements, the use of depression screening instruments has little or no impact on the detection, management and outcome of depression in PHC (Gilbody, Sheldon, & House, 2008). Screening tools are good but have to be supplemented with good clinical judgment (Patel, Simon, Chowdhary, Kaaya, & Araya, 2009) and should be part of a package of enhanced care. Otherwise implementing screening will increase cost without benefit (Gilbody, Sheldon, & Wessely, 2006).

2.2.5. The case of perinatal depression

The barriers to detection of depression in PHC that we have seen above also apply to perinatal depression. But because the perinatal period is unique it adds to the difficulty. Many believe that pregnancy is a time of joy for the mother and the whole family but this is not always the case. A study from Portugal found that knowledge barriers about the nature of the mental health problems and treatment options were some of the barriers to seeking help during the perinatal period (Fonseca, Gorayeb, & Canavarro, 2015). A qualitative study done in a HIC on female participants who gave birth in the last three years, who had psychological symptoms, revealed that women may be reluctant to disclose symptoms because a diagnosis of mental health problem might lead to stigma and loss of parental rights and some complained of negative experience with perinatal health care providers which affected communication (Byatt et al., 2013). In a study on postpartum women from Ethiopia, some of the frequently reported barriers to accessing depression care, among others, were thinking the problem would get better by itself, the woman wanting to solve the problem by herself, worry about distance and worry about cost of care (Azale et al., 2016).

Perinatal health care professionals from a high income country mentioned lack of resources, skills and confidence needed as a barrier to diagnose, refer and treat mothers with perinatal depression (Byatt et al., 2012).

Both depression and pregnancy share changes in appetite, sleep and energy as a common presentation and this overlap between symptoms of depression and symptoms associated with pregnancy may bias estimates of depression in studies of women of childbearing age (Matthey & Ross-Hamid, 2011; Yonkers, Smith, Gotman, & Belanger, 2009), which can also make diagnosis of depression in a clinical setting difficult.

Maternal health services also need to be structured to deliver continuing care. A study from primary maternal care facilities in Nigeria showed that there are major inadequacies in the organizational and administrative profile of facilities that works against the provision of quality chronic care (Ayinde et al., 2018) and this is the reality in most LMICs. The findings of a review article on midwife's role in perinatal mental health (Noonan, Doody, Jomeen, & Galvin, 2017) identified that midwives are constrained to provide care for women because of lack of referral options and the need for ongoing educational and organizational supports to confidently and optimally fulfill their role in perinatal mental health. The availability of access to appropriate resources and referral pathways may be important variables which influence midwives' confidence and practice (Noonan et al., 2017). In another study, limited access to mental health care and resources were identified as system-level barriers by perinatal health professionals (Byatt et al., 2012).

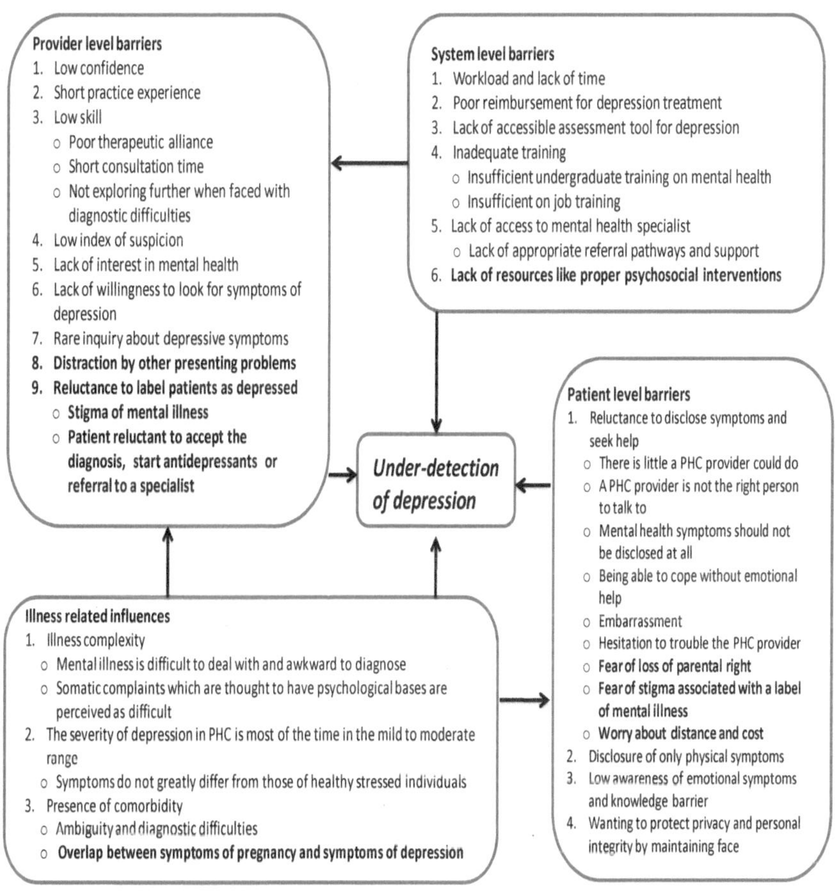

Figure 1: Conceptual framework for under-detection of depression in primary health care

2.3. Evaluation of approaches to overcome barriers to detection of depression

Improving the recognition of depression is the first step in increasing treatment accessibility and outcome. In the absence of active identification strategies, most individuals with depression will not seek or receive help. Different approaches have been tried to enable early recognition of depression. These are universal screening of patients in PHC using depression screening tools, providing appropriate training for PHC workers in the assessment and management of depression and integration of depression programs into existing health services using a task-sharing approach.

Universal screening within PHC was once seen as best practice to enable early recognition of depression in many settings (Milgrom & Gemmill, 2014). There are multiple depression screening tools available worldwide. Wherever possible, the screening tool to be used should be validated against a gold standard diagnostic assessment in the specific context in which it will be employed (Ali, Ryan, & De Silva, 2016).

Meta-analysis of studies from HICs suggested that universal screening may not necessarily be the most efficient method for case detection (Cuijpers, van Straten, van Schaik, & Andersson, 2009). Although screening questionnaires are a useful tool in PHC, they need to be supplemented with clinical judgment as positive predictive values (PPVs) of questionnaires compared with a diagnostic assessment, is mostly low at the optimal cut-off scores (Hanlon et al., 2015; Van Heyningen, Honikman, Tomlinson, Field, & Myer, 2018). The study from Ethiopia indicated that depression screening questionnaires do not have immediate applicability in routine clinical settings and further studies should evaluate the depression screening questionnaires utility within health system changes that support depression detection (Girma et al.,2013; Hanlon et al., 2015). Clear pathways of systematic follow up of all positive screening results with a diagnostic procedure and access to treatment are centrally important both for the clinical effectiveness of screening and for health system costs (Milgrom & Gemmill, 2014). Focusing on patients with severe symptoms and assessing those who scored very high on screening questionnaires using DSM depression criteria is thought to decrease the burden on

PHC workers by accurately identifying depressed patients most in need of treatment (Nease, Klinkman, & Volk, 2002).

Appropriate training for PHC workers in the assessment and management of depression is the first step to maximize usefulness while minimizing potential harms of universal screening (Milgrom & Gemmill, 2014). But there are questions on the benefit of isolated training-based approaches. A positive result from a study conducted in Malawi (Kauye, Jenkins, & Rahman, 2014) has not been replicated. Looking at the experience of five LMICs from the PRIME project, even though training of PHC workers on WHO's mhGAP has been very successful in decreasing the treatment gap for severe mental illness in the district (Hailemariam, Fekadu, Medhin, Prince, & Hanlon, 2019; Hanlon et al., 2020), it has been less successful for internalizing disorders like depression (Fekadu et al., 2017; Jenkins et al., 2013; Rathod et al., 2018). This calls for innovation of a novel approach to enhance detection (Fekadu et al., 2020).

The delivery of depression treatments should ideally be carried out through an integration of depression programs into existing health services with task-sharing by non-specialist health workers to deliver front-line care supervised by appropriately skilled mental health workers (Patel, Simon, Chowdhary, Kaaya, & Araya, 2009). Again, task-sharing is not an outright solution for overcoming under detection of depression in LMICs (Padmanathan & De Silva, 2013). In order for task-sharing interventions to be successful, other factors need to be considered. These include task-sharing workforces' distress level, their self-perceived level of competence, the acceptance of the workforce by other health care professionals and the incentives provided to ensure workforce retention (Padmanathan & De Silva, 2013). It is also important to have depression treatment services available as the availability of treatment services and referral system may encourage PHC workers to screen for depression if they know where they can refer cases to.

Paying attention to not only to the psychological but also to the somatic symptoms of depression also would help to improve recognition in PHC settings as somatic symptoms play an important role in the manifestation of depressive disorders in PHC users (Barkow et al., 2004). Another way to increase detection of depression in primary care is by reassessment and having patients followed by the same clinician longitudinally. Studies show that diagnosis of depression by PHC workers was improved with prospective examination of patients over an extended period rather than relying on a one-off assessment (Mitchell, Vaze, & Rao, 2009).

Chapter three: Methods

3.1. Study design

This study used qualitative data collection methods. The study had two parts.

1. In-depth interviews (IDIs) with women who were pregnant and identified with moderate to severe depression or major depressive disorder. The interviews tried to explore women's understanding of their symptoms, whether they have communicated the symptoms, how they communicated their difficulties to the PHC worker, and their expectations and perspectives on possible interventions.

2. Focus group discussions (FGDs) were conducted with PHC workers who work in the ANC clinics from where the pregnant women were recruited. The discussion included what they understand depression to be, focusing on perinatal depression, and what they consider appropriate interventions to be in such situations. The FGDs also explored possible reasons for lower rates of diagnosis of depression than expected in the ANC clinics.

3.2. Study area

The study was conducted in four rural health centres and a primary hospital, located in the Sodo district, which is about 100 km south of the capital, Addis Ababa, Ethiopia. Sodo district was selected for this study because its PHC workers have been trained on mhGAP-IG and the area was a trial site for integration of mental health care into PHC. Four health centres, out of eight health centres in the Sodo district, and the primary hospital were selected based on the high flow of women they serve on a daily basis in their ANC clinics.

3.3. Population

We had two types of participants in the study.

1. Pregnant women attending ANC clinics of the four health centres or the primary hospital in the Sodo district, diagnosed with moderate to severe depression by PHC workers OR diagnosed with MDD by the research psychiatrist after scoring 5 or above on the PHQ-9.
2. PHC workers working in the Sodo district health centres and the primary hospital ANC clinics, where pregnant women for the first part of the study were recruited.

3.4. Inclusion and exclusion criteria

1. Pregnant women

Inclusion criteria:

The included participants were pregnant women attending the ANC clinic in one of the four health centres or the primary hospital who were given a diagnosis of moderate to severe depression by a PHC worker OR of MDD by the research psychiatrist after scoring 5 and above on the screening PHQ-9.

The exclusion criteria used were:

- Are acutely unwell and need emergency treatment
- Are unable to converse in Amharic, the official federal language of Ethiopia
- Are unable to communicate for any reason
- Did not give consent

2. PHC workers

Consenting PHC workers working in ANC clinics of the primary hospital and the four health centres, where pregnant women for the first part of the study were recruited, were included in the FGD. In order to have a rich understanding of the challenges PHC workers face in recognizing depression in pregnant women, and to explore their perspectives on possible solutions, purposive sampling was used. I intentionally tried to select ANC PHC workers based on the objective of the study by including PHC workers from the primary hospital and from both rural and urban health centers. I also included participants who had previous training on mhGAP and participants who did not have prior mhGAP training. Their duration of clinical experience also varied.

3.5. Participant recruitment procedure

3.5.1. Part I of the study: In-depth interviews with pregnant women with depression

Stage I

1. In the four selected Sodo district health centres, PHQ-9 was administered by lay data collectors to all pregnant women when they come for their ANC evaluation. The lay data collectors had prior experience with administration of PHQ-9, as they have been working on the site as data collectors for other similar research projects. In addition they were given refresher training on the administration of PHQ-9 by the research psychiatrist.

   The PHQ-9 score was given to the PHC workers, who were then expected to assess those women who scored 5 or above on the PHQ-9 for moderate to severe depression. This step was expected to increase their detection of moderate to severe depression. Those women with a diagnosis of moderate to severe depression made by a PHC worker were invited for an in-depth interview.

2. Those pregnant women who scored high on PHQ-9 but who were not diagnosed as having moderate to severe depression by PHC workers were reassessed by the research psychiatrist. Pregnant women who were diagnosed as having MDD (which is equivalent to mhGAP's moderate to severe depression) by the research psychiatrist were invited for an in-depth interview (See Figure 2).

   In practice, after four weeks of screening, participant recruitment was much lower than expected. Women were not coming on the appointment date for interview or for reassessment by a research psychiatrist and those who scored 5 or above on PHQ-9 and who attended for reassessment were not diagnosed as having MDD.

Stage II

Following the lack of identification of pregnant women with MDD, a half day training was conducted on administration and scoring of PHQ-9 for PHC workers who work in ANC clinics of the four selected Sodo district health centres. Refresher training was also given to them on the depression module of mhGAP-IG. The PHC workers were then asked to do PHQ-9 screening for all women who come for ANC follow up and do the moderate to severe depression assessment as per mhGAP-IG for those women who scored 5 or above on the PHQ-9 screening (See Figure 3). This was done with the assumption that if the PHC workers carried out the PHQ-9 screening themselves, instead of data collectors, indirectly they will be starting the depression assessment process which was expected to improve detection. Over a one-month period, there were a few women who scored 5 and above on PHQ-9 but none were diagnosed as having moderate to severe depression.

Stage III

We expected a higher number of pregnant women with depression from the four health centres based on the number of women they see in a day and from the prevalence estimates we had from previous studies done in the same area. Since the above two participant recruitment methods were not very successful, we decided to include an additional recruitment method to the ones described above.

We added the district's primary hospital to the four selected health centres as a study site. PHQ-9 was administered by the lay data collectors to all pregnant women when they come for their ANC evaluation. The screening went on for one month. After their ANC evaluation those women who scored 5 or above on PHQ-9, but who did not receive a diagnosis of moderate to severe depression by the PHC worker, were sent to a Mental Health Focal Person (MHFP) of the respective health centre or hospital for assessment of depression. In the primary hospital the MHFP is a psychiatric nurse but in the health centres these are PHC workers who are appointed as a focal person for mental health. MHFPs of health centres tend to see more patients with mental health problems but they do not have additional training on mental health other than mhGAP-IG. Those women who were assessed as having moderate to severe depression or MDD by the MHFP or were diagnosed with moderate to severe depression by a PHC worker working in the ANC clinics were contacted and invited to take part in the study by the research psychiatrist (See Figure 4).

3.5.2. Part II of the study: FGDs with PHC workers working in the ANC clinics

As mentioned above, PHC workers from the ANC clinics of the four health centres and the primary hospital were included in one of the two FGDs, after they gave consent.

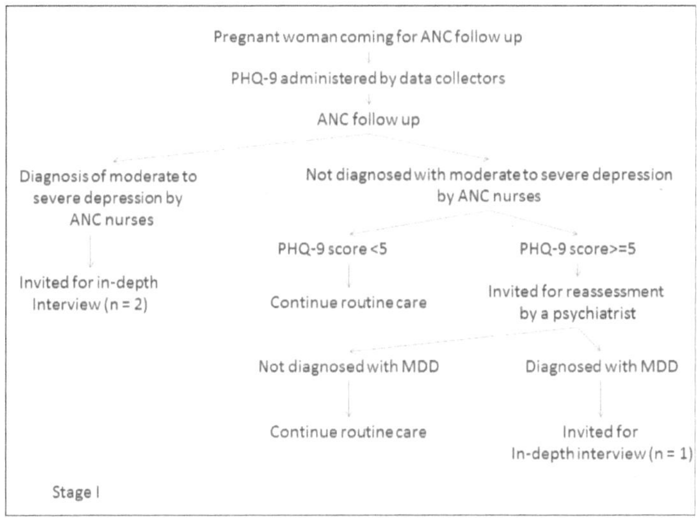

Figure 2: Stage I of IDI participant recruitment procedure

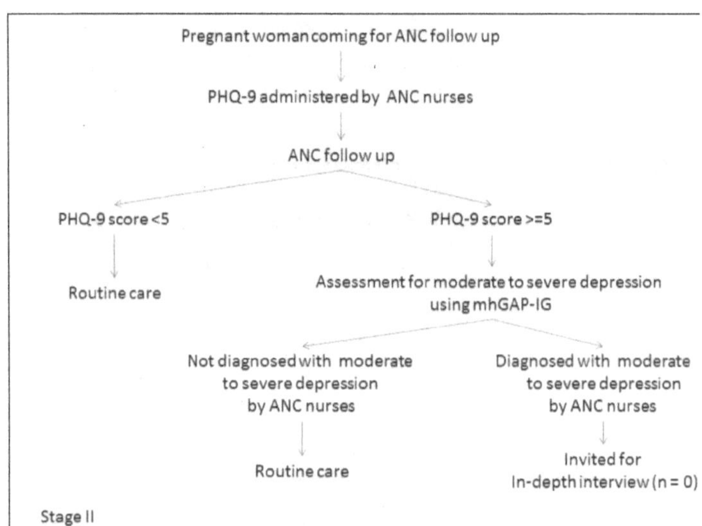

Figure 3:Stage II of IDI participant recruitment procedure

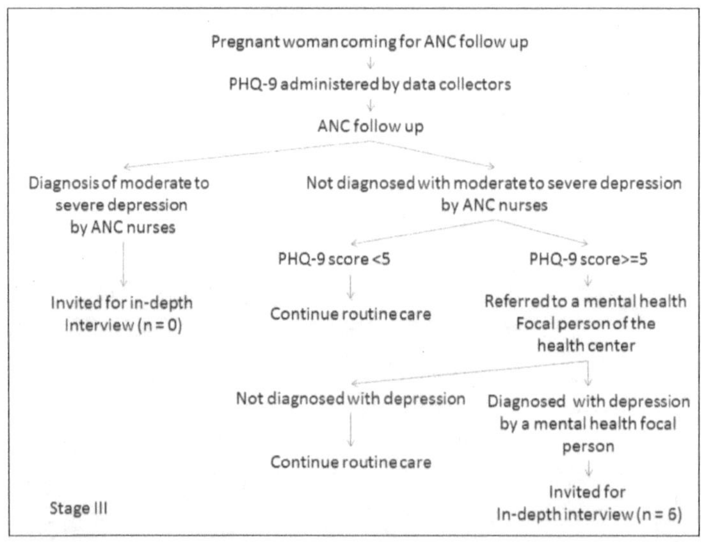

Figure 4: Stage III of IDI participant recruitment procedure

3.6. Sample size

The aim was to recruit a total of twelve women with a diagnosis of moderate to severe depression in the first part of the study, but data saturation determined the final number. I decided data saturation had been achieved when the new in-depth interviews were repeating what was expressed earlier and no new information was being discovered. This indicated that conducting further interviews was unnecessary.

A total of 14 ANC PHC workers, from the four health centres and the primary hospital were invited to participate in the FGDs.

3.7. Data collection tools

1. Socio-demographic characteristics:

Women's self-report of age, educational level, marital status, employment status, gestational age, any problem identified in the current pregnancy, and other indicators of socio-economic status (Appendix 3.1 and 3.2).

ANC PHC workers' age, sex, educational background, work place, duration of practice, experience working in ANC clinic and training on mhGAP (Appendix 3.3)

2. Depression diagnosis

   2.1. Diagnosis of moderate to severe depression by ANC PHC workers using the mhGAP-IG

   2.2. Patient Health Questionnaire, 9 item version (PHQ-9)

   The PHQ-9 is a brief self-report questionnaire designed as a screening tool for depression in primary care. The PHQ-9 has nine items and can be used to rate symptom severity and monitor change over time (Kroenke & Spitzer, 2002; Kroenke, Spitzer, & Williams, 2001). It has already been translated into Amharic, the official language of Ethiopia, and this Amharic version has been validated in clinical settings (Girma, 2013; Gelaye et al., 2013; Hanlon et al., 2015) (Appendix 4.1 and 4.2). In a sample of pregnant women, at an optimal cut off score of greater than or equal to four, the PHQ-9 had a sensitivity of 86.7%, specificity of

80.4%, PPV of 15.1% and negative predictive value (NPV) of 99.3%. At a cut off score of greater than or equal to five, it had a sensitivity of 66.7%, specificity of 89.3%, PPV of 20.2% and NPV of 98.5% (Girma, 2013).

The reason for administering the PHQ-9 was to increase the detection of moderate to severe depression by PHC workers and to help screen patients who had a high probability of having MDD, since a psychiatrist cannot assess all women.

2.3. The research psychiatrist conducted a clinical interview to screen for the presence of MDD, using DSM 5 diagnostic criteria, for those who scored high on PHQ-9 but were not diagnosed as having moderate to severe depression by the PHC workers.

3. In-depth interviews were conducted with the pregnant women who were diagnosed with moderate to severe depression by a PHC worker OR MDD by the research psychiatrist. Numbers were not pre-set for each type of participant.

   A guide for the in-depth interview was developed to assess understanding and communication of symptoms by women diagnosed to have moderate to severe depression OR MDD. This in-depth interview guide was used for the interviews (Appendix 5.1 and 5.2).

4. Focus group discussions (FGDs) with PHC workers (Appendix 5.3). FGDs were audio recorded and notes were taken.

   A FGD guide was developed and used during the discussions. The FGD guide explored possible reasons for low detection of depression in the ANC clinics and potential approaches to solving the problems identified from the first part of the study.

3.8. Data collection procedures

PHQ-9 was administered to all pregnant women by data collectors or ANC clinic PHC workers. A detailed contact address was taken for those women who scored five or above on PHQ-9 or for those who were diagnosed with moderate to severe depression. These women were contacted by the researcher and were given detailed information about the study and asked for their consent to take part (Appendix 1 and 2). Written informed consent was obtained after the information was read to the potential participant in Amharic and a copy of the information sheet had been given to them. Only those who gave written informed consent, either by putting their signature or fingerprint on the consent form, were included in the interviews. For those potential participants who were not literate, a witness was present during the informed consent process and both the witness and the participant put their signature or fingerprint on the consent form. Socio-demographic data was collected for all women included in the study.

The in-depth interviews were conducted with pregnant women with a diagnosis of moderate to severe depression or MDD using the in-depth interview guide. All interviews took place in a separate room and in a place where privacy and confidentiality were maintained. The interviews were audio-recorded and notes were taken.

After summarising the findings from the first part of the study, two FGDs were carried out with the health care providers of the ANC clinics from the four health centres and the primary hospital. In addition to further exploration of reasons for non-detection of depression as expressed by the PHC workers, there were discussions about how care can be improved at the PHC level for pregnant women with moderate to severe depression.

During the in-depth interviews and FGDs, I was conscious of my bias as a psychiatrist and tried my best not to influence participants' response by being neutral to whatever was coming up during the process and exploring further without suggesting anything. Since all women and PHC workers were aware that I was a medical doctor and a psychiatrist, it might have possibly affected how they responded during interviews and discussions.

3.9. Data analysis

A framework approach to qualitative data analysis was used. The framework method is a systematic way of analyzing qualitative data. It analyzes data by case and by code, and the defining feature is the matrix output of rows (cases), columns (codes) and cells of summarized data (Ritchie, Lewis, Nicholls, & Ormston, 2013). Built into the structure and process of the framework approach is the ability to compare data across as well as within individual cases with ease (Gale, Heath, Cameron, Rashid, & Redwood, 2013). The conceptual framework developed during the literature review formed the basis for the analytical framework used for data analysis.

The recorded data from the in-depth interviews and FGDs were first transcribed verbatim and then translated into English. As data collection proceeded, the transcripts were read and re-read to get to know and understand the data. Analysis was carried out using the translated English versions.

The coding process started with open coding, where initial descriptive codes were applied to the data. I and another psychiatrist independently coded the first two interviews. This initial coding was followed by a discussion on differences noticed and agreement was reached before the rest of the transcripts were coded. In the process, a code book was developed.

After coding of all interviews and FGDs, I categorized all relevant information based on the conceptual framework (Figure 1). I started with pre-set categories but also dealt with emerging themes. Themes and patterns were identified. After this step, I identified patterns and connections within and between categories, analyzed their relative importance and relationships. Finally, I tried to explain the findings and what we have learned.

I tried to ensure rigor by clearly showing how we came to such conclusions and involving all research members in the analysis process. I used computer software - OpenCode during the process.

3.10. Ethical considerations

Ethical permission was obtained from University of Cape Town (HREC REF: 515/2015) and the Institutional Review Board of the College of Health Sciences, Addis Ababa University (Protocol number: 048/15/psych) (Appendix 6.1 and 6.2).

Those women who were diagnosed as having MDD by the research psychiatrist and who had not received any kind of intervention from the PHC worker were advised to see a nearby psychiatric nurse. The location and how to access the service was explained to the participants in detail. In addition, participating women were given psychoeducation about their condition and were told that they could contact the research psychiatrist using the contact address provided in the information sheet if they had additional questions or needed help.

Only those health care providers and pregnant women who gave written, informed consent were included in the study. The consent process, as well as the discussion, was held in Amharic so only those who could speak Amharic were invited to participate in the study. The information and consent was administered by the research psychiatrist, who does not work in the health centre, to make it easier for the pregnant women to refuse participation if they did not wish to take part in the study. Participants were clearly told that choosing not to take part in the study would not disadvantage them in any way. For all pregnant women, information was given, consent was obtained, socio-demographic and other data were collected and interviews took place in private rooms. Interviews were audio-recorded with participants consent. All participants were reimbursed for their time and transport cost. All participants were informed that they could withdraw from the study at any time if they wished to. Recordings from interviews and discussions as well as other field notes and questionnaires did not contain any identifying data. We made sure that nobody, except the principal investigator and research advisors, knew that particular information belonged to a particular person. All data were kept in a secure location which only the researchers could access. All audio-recordings were deleted after data analysis.

Chapter four: Results

4.1. Socio-demographic characteristics of In-depth interview participants

A total of nine women were included in the first part of the study (See Table 1). Their age ranged from 21 to 37 years. Four of the participants were able to read and write (most attending primary education) and five were illiterate, with either a very low level of formal education (grade one or two) or no education at all. For the pregnant women, the gestational age ranged from three months to nine months. One woman was six weeks postpartum at the time of interview. For all participants, the current pregnancy was not their first.

Table 1: Description of the socio-demographic characteristics of the perinatal women (n= 9)

			Number
Age in years	20-24		2
	25-29		5
	30-34		1
	35-39		1
Literacy	Literate		4
	Illiterate		5
Education type	Formal (Grades completed)	1-4	3
		5-8	2
		9-10	1
	No education		3
Marital status	Married		7
	Separated		2
Residence place	Urban		2
	Rural		7
Occupation	Housewife		1
	Farmer		4
	Merchant		3
	Daily laborer		1
Subjective relative wealth (relative to others in same village [kebele])	Similar		3
	Less		6
Perinatal status	First trimester		1
	Second trimester		1
	Third trimester		6
	Postpartum		1
Number of living children	One		3
	Two		3
	Three		1
	Four		2

4.2. Clinical characteristics of In-depth interview participants

The participants in the first part of the study were recruited from one urban health centre (Kella), one rural health centre (Adele) and one primary hospital (Buei). No participant was recruited from two of the four health centres (Tiya and Wella Wella Wedesha) used to recruit participants, as there were none who fulfilled the inclusion criteria. The women's PHQ-9 total score ranged from 6 to 12. Only two participants received a diagnosis of moderate to severe depression from primary care workers in the ANC clinics. The research psychiatrist diagnosed three participants as having major depressive disorder, one with somatic symptom disorder, one with an anxiety disorder and four women with no current psychiatric diagnosis (although two had a history of depression) as set out in Table 2.

Table 2: Clinical information of pregnant women who participated in the study (n = 9)

Code	Health institution	PHQ-9 score	Diagnosis of depression		Diagnosis by researcher (Psychiatrist)	Remark
			ANC staff	Mental health focal person		
101	Primary hospital	6	No	Yes	No MDD	Dissociative symptoms and obsessions, possible personality disorder
102	Primary hospital	8	No	Yes	Somatic symptom disorder	
103	Primary hospital	12	No	Yes	MDD	
201	Urban health centre	7	No	N/A	Currently does not have depression	Has epilepsy, had history of depression and psychosis secondary to epilepsy and alcohol use disorder
202	Urban health centre	7	Yes	N/A	MDD	
203	Urban health centre	6	No	Yes	Anxiety disorder	
204	Urban health centre	11	No	Yes	MDD	
301	Rural health centre	8	Yes	N/A	No MDD	Reported that head position of fetus is not correct
302	Rural health centre	11	No	Yes	Currently does not have depression	Had previous history of depression

MDD: Major Depressive Disorder, N/A: Not Applicable

4.3. Symptoms endorsed on PHQ-9 for each of the women

During screening, the participating women endorsed a combination of emotional, physical and cognitive symptoms on the PHQ-9. Table 3 sets out the symptoms endorsed on the PHQ-9 by individual woman.

*Table 3: Symptoms endorsed on PHQ-9 for each woman (n=8)**

Participant ID	Little interest or pleasure in doing things	Feeling down, depressed, or hopeless	Trouble falling or staying asleep, or sleeping too much†	Feeling tired or having little energy†	Poor appetite or overeating†	Feeling bad about yourself - or that you are a failure or have let yourself or your family down	Trouble concentrating on things	Moving or speaking so slowly Or the opposite - being so fidgety or restless	Thoughts that you would be better off dead or of hurting yourself in some way
MDD									
103		x	x	x	x	x			x
202	X	x	x	x	x				
204	X	x	x	x	x		x		
No MDD									
101	X	x	x	x			x	X	
102		x	x	x	x				x
201	X	x	x	x	x		x		
301	X		x	x	x		x	X	
302	X	x	x	x	x		x		x

*PHQ-9 scorning form couldn't be located for one participant, ID 203

†Overlapping symptoms of depression and pregnancy

4.4. Focus group discussion participants' characteristics

Twelve ANC clinic PHC workers were included in the two FGDs. They were from one urban (Kella) and two rural (Adele and Wella Wella Wedesha) health centres and the primary hospital. PHC workers from Tiya heath centre were invited to participate in the FGDs but were not included because they did not show up for the discussion. Ten of the participants were female. All of the participants were midwives by profession and had a chance to work in the ANC clinics in the past one year. Half of them had undergone mhGAP training at least once during their practice. See Table 4.

Table 4: Socio-demographic characteristics of PHC workers who participated in the study (n = 12)

Demographic characteristics of PHC workers		Number
Age in years	20-24	3
	25-29	8
	30-34	1
Gender	Male	2
	Female	10
Health Centre/Hospital	Buei	2
	Kella	6
	Adele	1
	Wula Wula Wedesa	3
Educational Background	Midwife	12
Experience working in ANC clinic in the past one year	Yes	12
	No	0
Total duration of practice as a clinician	<1 year	3
	1 – 5 years	8
	>5 years	1
Previous training on mhGAP	Yes	6
	No	6

4.5. Themes on under detection of depression in pregnant women

It was evident that women were not sharing the psychological distress they had with ANC PHC workers. Similarly, ANC PHC workers were not routinely assessing pregnant women for depression, even if they were potentially at risk. The framework analysis resulted in the generation of four themes and ten sub-themes exploring barriers to detection and diagnosis of depression in the ANC clinics.

4.5.1. Client level barriers

Reluctance to disclose symptoms and seek help

Eight out of nine participating perinatal women were reluctant to disclose the non-physical symptoms they had to the ANC PHC worker and as a result did not share their distress at their ANC follow up. This happened irrespective of whether or not they thought they had an illness. The reasons given included not even considering mentioning it:

"It never occurred to me..." ID 201

"...I haven't thought of it." ID 202

Whereas other women thought that there was little ANC PHC worker could do.

"I did not know that they know anything and I thought that they could not help me and I stayed silent." ID 302

"I don't know what good it can do to tell them." ID 203

Interviewer:	*"What type of problems can they [ANC PHC workers] help with?"*
Interviewee:	*"When people are stressed with labour or they get sick, with God, they will help. When people have physical illness like typhoid or if there is an emergency labour then they would help."*
Interviewer:	*"Who do you think would help if the problem is mental illness?"*
Interviewee:	*"I would not think of it [I don't think they can help]." ID 201*

One participant did not want to disclose because of hopelessness.

Interviewee:	*"I didn't want to live at the time. I thought, if I die, then let it be. But if I wanted to live, I would have asked [for help]."*
Interviewer:	*"You didn't ask [for help] because you wanted to die at the time?"*
Interviewee:	*"I was angry at his [husband's] house. I caused pain to my mother and brothers. I thought that if I die they could live properly, and my mother would raise my children actively, and that my brothers would live properly. That's what I thought around me [at that time]." ID 302*

Another woman did not want to disclose her symptoms, worrying about what would happen as a result.

Interviewee:	*"It's like I told you before, I am scared of getting injections and that's why."*
Interviewer:	*"If you tell them [ANC PHC workers] the problem?"*
Interviewee:	*"Yes, if I tell them the problem they will give me an injection."*
Interviewer:	*"And that will restart the old illness [described as a spirit]?"*
Interviewee:	*"It would start my old illness [the spirit] again and will put me in a problem." ID 101*

One woman felt that, if she shared mental health problem during ANC visits, her complaints may not be accepted and feared that disclosure might change how the health worker treated her.

"... I don't think that they [ANC PHC workers] would accept it. I think if we were to tell them [the stress we have], they would have bad attitude toward us." ID 203

Even though it was raised in relation with heavy alcohol use, another woman mentioned that she lied about her alcohol use when asked at the OPD, where she had a follow-up consultation for epilepsy. The reason she gave was fear of being judged.

Interviewee: "Yes I hid it [my drinking] because he [the clinician] is a neighbor."
Interviewer: "What is it that holds you back from speaking?"
Interviewee: "I don't want to tell. It is a secret."
Interviewer: "What do you think will happen if you tell?"
Interviewee: "I think they will say she always drinks."
Interviewer: "You think they will see you negatively? Or judge you?"
Interviewee: "I think that they will look down on me, saying that she drinks and that's why I hid it." ID 201

One woman (diagnosed with somatic symptom disorder) spoke of her experience of repeatedly telling PHC ANC staff about the problems she had, which were mostly physical. She had been asking them to refer her to a hospital for better evaluation as she was convinced that she had a problem. As seen from this quote, the woman was not satisfied with the physical interventions offered by the PHC workers.

"I went there [health centre ANC clinic] asked them to give me [a referral]. I was feeling tired. I did not do anything with that thing. I had a huge change, what is this? I went to Buei [the hospital] because I wanted x-ray [ultrasound] and to see my child's position in my belly and see the sickness in it. In [the health centre] they said to wait till seven month and two weeks and that they would give me a referral. They said till then I don't have anything to worry about. I told them I had poor appetite, I am sick and I told them that when I go to them they give me seven injections and a hundred and thirty pills. I said to them that they only tell me to take these pills and eat this... and I have a poor appetite for food and I am getting tired." ID 102

What is thought to be the cause of symptoms

Participating women talked about reasons they thought were causes for the symptoms or difficulties they had. Except for one mother, who was strongly convinced of having an illness, all listed multiple possible reasons as a cause. Five of the nine participants thought what they had was an illness, and in addition they mentioned relationship problems, financial difficulties, unwanted pregnancy or the pregnancy itself and/or bad spirit (Satan) as causes.

Interviewee: *"Regardless, if I have [other life problems] or not, if I am healthy I will work. My problem is with my health."*
Interviewer: *"So you think that there is no cause for it?"*
Interviewee: *"I think the reason is that I just think by myself and worry, I say that I am less than them....I say to myself how can I be less than other people. If it is because of this or on its own....it confused me....I think it is an illness but other than that I don't know."*
Interviewer: *"What kind of illness do you think it is?"*
Interviewee: *"I think it's an illness that stresses me. What do I know?" ID 203*

One woman was not sure whether what she experienced was an illness but feared it might lead to one.

Interviewee: *"I don't know [what caused it]. I think it's because of anger, when I have words [argument] with my husband and I get angry." "I don't know I just thought I might be ill."*
Interviewer: *"What kind of illness did you think it was, physical or related to the mind?"*
Interviewee: *"I fear it might be illness of the mind."*
Interviewer: *"You think it is?"*
Interviewee: *"Yes that's what I fear." ID 101*

Three of the nine women thought what they had was not an illness and said it was because of financial difficulties, marital problems, bewitchment and/or epilepsy.

> *"It's [I have these symptoms] because I don't work, I'm not working and not meeting with people. When I worked at the market, I had lots of friends. And I'll talk to them if they were there and I would get in [home] at night. I did not lose hope but now I don't like sitting with people and talking to them.... I don't consider it as an illness, it's when I face problems. I don't think [of it as an illness]." ID 103*

> *"I did not know anything like this [illness] before, like I told you I think it was someone's doing [bewitchment] but I did not know....It was someone's hand. But I got traditional medication and thank God I am better now." ID 201*

All women, except one, said their symptoms are not caused by pregnancy. Their arguments for it were; their symptoms started before the current pregnancy and their current symptoms are different from what they have experienced in their previous pregnancies.

Interviewer: *"do you think it [the problem you have] has something to do with the pregnancy?"*
Interviewee: *"No, it even was there before [my pregnancy]" ID 301*

Interviewer: *"Do you think the pregnancy is the cause [for your problem]?"*
Interviewee: *"[No] I had it in the past too."*
Interviewer: *"But is this feeling of tiredness not part of your pregnancy?"*
Interviewee: *"Yes."*
Interviewer: *"It is related to that?"*
Interviewee: *"No, I don't think it is. I wouldn't have lost this much [energy] at other times [previous pregnancies]" ID 203*

Interviewee: *"The difficulty is expected. But I worry about what will happen to me. This heaviness is expected, isn't it difficult to carry a baby [in your belly]?"*
Interviewer: *"It's difficult, that's right, it's difficult."*
Interviewee: *"But I have been polluted with this sickness. Why am I getting [this much] tired now? I have had children before." ID 102*

Interviewer: *"We think that most of the time when pregnancy starts there is nausea but through time it gets better."*
Interviewee: *"This is different."*
Interviewer: *"It's different?"*
Interviewee: *"Yes."*
Interviewer: *"You told me earlier that you feel tired, but when there is pregnancy there is also being tired, is it different from your past pregnancy?"*
Interviewee: *"Yes." ID 204*

What is thought to help with symptoms

When women were asked what they thought would help them with the problems they had, five out of nine women mentioned interventions that did not involve modern medical treatment. These include use of traditional medication, praying to God, holy water treatment and improvement in financial and marital difficulties.

Interviewer: *"When problems like this occur, what do you think could be the solution? for anger and sadness?"*
Interviewee: *"Before I thought it was holy water."*
Interviewer: *"They say that it is holy water?"*
Interviewee: *"Like before, I only think it's holy water."*
Interviewer: *"You think that's the solution?"*
Interviewee: *"I think it's only that....I think it's holy water, that's the solution and nothing else." ID 101*

Interviewer: *"When these problems existed and were at their worst, what did you think would have helped them? Did you think if you did something, you could get rid of these problems or make them better in some way?"*
Interviewee: *"I did not think anything. I only prayed to God to lift it and to make me equal with my friends. I prayed 'please take what you have brought'."*
Interviewer: *"Are you saying that praying helps?"*
Interviewee: *"Yes I think that prayer helps me..... I prayed to God saying 'I have no father or mother, please take what you have brought'. I prayed that morning and night and I prayed and I prayed. I took holy water for some time and I got better." ID 201*

Interviewer: *"Okay, in your understanding what can help with these problems? When you feel angry, stressed or feel like going. How do you think that the things that come to your mind can be fixed?"*
Interviewee: *"I don't know anything."*
Interviewer: *"... do you think it will get better as the day goes by?"*
Interviewee: *"Yes."*
Interviewer: *"What could make it better?"*
Interviewee: *"When you work and reach where you want to get, you [what you feel] may change. If I was not like this [pregnant and not working because of it and as a result have no income] I would go to the market and [make money and I will change" ID 103*

Four out of nine women said they think they might get a solution for the problems they have from a modern medical treatment center. Despite this, women did not share their emotional difficulties with ANC PHC workers. This was because they were considering mental health departments/psychiatric clinic rather than ANC clinics to report these symptoms.

Interviewer: *"Have you ever thought yours may be an illness, like a disease?"*
Interviewee: *"Yes I have. I say I need to go for evaluation at a higher center, when I experience it."*
Interviewer: *"When you say 'when I experience it' which experience are you referring to?"*
Interviewee: *"The depression and the like."*
Interviewer: *"Good! So you want to get evaluated thinking it may be an illness? ..... When you were thinking of having high level evaluation, where were you thinking [of going]?"*
Interviewee: *"No, Butajira [referral hospital where there is a psychiatry clinic]"*
Interviewer: *"Going to Butajira .... hospital and telling them?"*
Interviewee: *"yes" ID 202*

Interviewer: *"Do you think that medical care can help [with the problems you have]"?*

Interviewee: *"Yes."*
Interviewer: *"What type of medical care can help?"*
Interviewee: *"Something like a pill or injection."*
Interviewer: *"Do you think they would be able to give you medical care, the people that were treating you during the pregnancy? Do you think they have a solution for this?"*
Interviewee: *"I don't think that."*
Interviewer: *"You don't think so? But who do you think might have a solution for this? You said the pills or shots [might be able to help you], you said that correct?"*
Interviewee: *"Yes."*
Interviewer: *"Who do you think can do [give you] that?*
Interviewee: *"It could be a doctor or something."*
Interviewer: *"Yes, but doctors [health workers] work there [at the ANC clinic] correct?"*
Interviewee: *"Yes."*
Interviewer: *"What type of doctor do you think it is? If you had to guess?"*
Interviewee: *"What do I know? Just a doctor."*
Interviewer: *"When you say doctor, are they different from the ones that treat you for your pregnancy?"*
Interviewee: *"If I find someone better than them." ID 203*

4.5.2. Provider level barriers

Not asking about depressive symptoms

That the ANC health workers did not ask about depressive symptoms was a recurring concern in almost all interviews. Participating women said that they expected to be asked in order for them to tell the health worker about any non-physical symptoms. Participating women also reported that they were not asked about emotional symptoms.

> *"They tell me to return after a month or two ... but they don't ask me 'is there any problem? How are you inside? What are you thinking?' ..." ID 202*

> *"I told them [data collectors the symptoms I have] because they asked, but what could I say without being asked?" ID 103*

A woman was not assessed for depression, even though she was convinced of having mental health problems and disclosed that to the PHC worker.

> *"They don't ask me ..... when I told them I have a mental problem, they say no. They think that I had Typhoid and Typhus. Nothing else, they say I caught Typhus" ID 203*

One woman indicated that even if she feared receiving injections, deep down she wanted to share her problem with PHC workers but wasn't asked.

> *Interviewee:* *"... but I wanted to tell [my problems] to them [the ANC PHC worker] deep inside. If I didn't want to tell them, I wouldn't have told them [the data collectors]."*
> *Interviewer:* *"You told the others [data collectors] because they asked you?"*
> *Interviewee:* *"Yes, if I really didn't want to tell, I could have said I have nothing and would have returned home." ID 101*

Most ANC PHC workers, during the FGDs, admitted that they do not routinely ask pregnant women about depressive symptoms, thus supporting the pregnant women's narratives.

> *"These [what the women said] are right, we have experienced it. To share my experience, when she comes in I would directly check the ANC checkup, not if she feels depressed. I may ask how she is doing or if she feels something but other than that we would not make it specific and ask them if she feels depressed or if there is something that is stressing her, we wouldn't ask such details ... ... Yes, most of the time they are not asked but some of us might ask." FGD participant ID 10*

FGD participants from the rural health centres expected women to open up and report the emotional difficulties they have when they ask them a general question "how are you doing/feeling?" and thought that this was a good screening question for depression. These ANC PHC workers were surprised to learn that the women said they were not asked about their emotional problems.

> *FGD participant ID 1:* *"I mean when we question them most of the time we don't ask them if they are depressed or stressed out. We will just ask them the overall conditions like that... thinking that they will explain everything to us; if they are sad, if they feel any other thing... that's what we ask them. At that time they will tell us."*
> *Interviewer:* *"So are you surprised about the fact that they didn't say anything?"*
> *FGD participant ID 1:* *"Yes"*

FGD participants, after hearing what participating women said during in-depth interviews, said ANC PHC workers should carry out a holistic assessment and not only focus on pregnancy follow ups. They proposed asking depression specific questions in order to assess mothers. In addition, they reported that ANC PHC workers should encourage mothers to talk about mental health problems they have and that providers should ensure privacy and maintaining confidentiality.

> *"We need to ask the whole situation, not only about the pregnancy. Telling her [a mother] that she can get the service here at the clinic, if she feels anything and also about the future situation too. As a health professional it is our responsibility to perform those tasks. Even if our level [in mental health knowledge] differs we need to take the mother's history so it she can tell us her whole situation and to be able to ask her history properly. And also improving the confidentiality so that one person won't pass history of one patient to another person and by doing that you can assure them their problem is safe with one person. With those things I think we can improve." FGD participant ID 10*

Reluctance to disclose diagnosis to patients

During the first FGD with rural health centre ANC PHC workers, reluctance to disclose a diagnosis of depression to women was mentioned because of fear of adding stress on the women. For most participants, it was not reported from experience as they never had identified cases.

FGD participant ID 3: "I don't think that it [telling a woman that she has depression] will be good for her"
Interviewer: "Okay so have you told her [the women you identified as having depression] at that time?"
FGD participant ID 3: "No, I didn't tell her"
Interviewer: "Okay so you haven't told her directly that the symptoms she was telling you were because of an illness named depression because you think it wouldn't be good for her?"
FGD participant ID 3: "Yes....maybe that mother will still worry, if we tell her after she comes here she will stress about it even more"

Interviewer: "[if you come across a woman with depression] will you not tell that she has this type of illness?"
FGD participant ID 2: "No, I will not tell her"
Interviewer: "Why don't you want to do so?"
FGD participant ID 2: "The reason that I don't want, is because, if I tell her that, she will worry that she has this illness and she might think of getting treatment for that. She might worry saying that I told her she has an illness."
Interviewer: "Because you think that it might add more stress for her?"
FGD participant ID 2: "Yes, so that it will not add more stress for her. Because I can easily

tell her to perform other tasks [that can relax her]"

"We never have depressed women in our ANC clinics"

ANC PHC workers from the rural health centres, during FGD one, were strongly convinced that the reason for not diagnosing pregnant women with depressive disorder was because there were none in their clinics. They mentioned that such women [with mental illness] are mostly seen in the general out-patient clinics (the 'OPD') which are not specific for perinatal women. They reported that it would not be difficult for them to identify and diagnose a woman with depression if one came to their clinic. Participants were supporting one another when discussing this topic as can be seen in the following quotes.

> *"Maybe there are many mentally ill people in our area. Even if there are, there are none that came to ANC, we didn't get the chance to see them. From what I know there are many mothers that came to OPD with a separate card to get a treatment with problems [mental health problems] but the ones that came for treatment in ANC don't have the problem that much." FGD participant ID 3*

> *"Those who describe such illness are the ones that come to the OPD, but those cases who present here [at the ANC] they won't tell us since they don't have it, but if there was any they would have said something." FGD participant ID 3*

> *"There are lots of them [with mental illness] that come here just like she [another participant] mentioned it. There are children, young and older people that come here but mothers do not have that..."FGD participant ID 2*

> *"They [women with mental illness] are not there at the ANC clinic where we work at. But they might be there at the OPD clinic... I haven't come across [depressed] pregnant women." FGD participant ID 1*

During the second FGD, which had ANC PHC workers from urban sites (Kella health centre and Buei Hospital), depressed women not being in their clinics did not come up. Instead multiple system level factors were raised as barriers to identifying depression in pregnant women in the ANC clinics.

4.5.3. System level barriers

Setting not conducive for depression assessment

Several system level barriers emerged mostly during the FGD with urban ANC PHC workers. Most PHC workers working in the ANC clinics acknowledged the difficulty in identifying cases and mentioned a number of challenges. Workload and lack of time, lack of resources, like separate rooms to see women privately, and perinatal women being followed up by different PHC workers over time were all mentioned as contributing factors for under-detection of depression in their ANC clinics.

> *"...and as it was stated earlier in order to guide and also the privacy, at the same time, those are needed. ... Specially in health centres the room that we use, it might be one or two, and if the professionals are many then we would be two or three [in a single room]. But if, for example, there are a lot of cases, in order to finish [quickly] in the same case one person might measure BP and another will clerk. When it is like that in order to draw their [women's] attention and in terms of privacy there might be a problem." FGD participant ID 5*

> *FGD participant ID 12: "Yeah it is something like that [our clinic is a difficult place to be seen]. Most of the time it is not a place that protects privacy"*
> *Interviewer: "Do many people get treated at the clinic at the same time?"*
> *FGD participant ID 12: "No, it is not like that. But there are a lot of cases – it's not a place that we can work alone".*
> *Interviewer: "So there is a case load?"*
> *FGD participant ID 12: "Yeah and there is shortage of rooms. It is not independent by itself [not separate for one PHC worker]"*
> *Interviewer: "The rooms are small so they might not also say anything?"*
> *FGD participant ID 12: "They won't say anything"*

> *"So relating with depression even one person at ANC first can see it. So around this area a mother would prefer to see a professional that knows her case and that saw her in the ANC for the first time [previously]. But that's not possible here since she will meet new person [ANC PHC worker] every time she came here for checkup, so she wouldn't be free to talk about it. But if it is a person that she is used to and is friendly, she would prefer to talk to that person." FGD participant ID 5*

Participants from the first FGD said that caseload and lack of time were not considered as a problem in their health centres.

Interviewer: *"So sometimes it is the professionals that claim about having a lot of things to do and they don't have time or they don't have much time to ask the necessary questions. So have you experienced such kinds of challenges in the system which makes it difficult for you to treat pregnant women with mental illness?*

FGD participant ID 1: "No there isn't"

Inadequate training on psychiatric disorders

Lack of training on psychiatric illnesses, absence of refresher training and inadequate follow-up following mhGAP trainings were problems described by FGD participants. These were one of the challenges mentioned as a barrier to providing quality mental health care to pregnant women during ANC checkups.

> *"There is nothing much that I can say. Since we didn't even get the training properly we were not able to focus on it [mental health]." FGD participant ID 12*

FGD participant ID 9: *"...we are not giving attention to the situation [mental illness]....The mother, the pregnancy, and also on the child, that's where I focus at the clinic. I suggest if we get trained and work"*

Interviewer: *"Do you think that you are able to care [for the mothers] better [if you get training on psychiatric disorders]?*

FGD participant ID 9: *"Yes"*

> *"It was better when we were at school because we were taking the course [Psychiatry].... But now most of us, we forgot about it. Because, as to me, I haven't taken mhGAP training. And the second one is that we focus on our profession [midwifery] and we don't have the habit of reading." FGD participant ID 10*

> *"There might be some updated things. For example we took the training back then [2014] and there might be things that are updated. We don't know about those since we took the training only once" FGD participant ID 11*

> *"What I want to add is what number eight has already touched on, which I mean most of the time what we took in terms of training... around the time where we took the training, we work properly but after some time we decrease doing it. It needs a follow up. Most of the time, what we have got through training needs a follow up like where did it reach [how many are detected or treated]." FGD participant ID 5*

There was a strong emphasis on the need for training. They suggested that all PHC workers who work at maternal and child (MCH) clinics should be trained on mental illnesses. The importance of having follow-ups and supervision following training was discussed. Sharing experience from those who have better expertise on the area was mentioned as one way of improving PHC workers skill on depression assessment.

> *"If there is an update every time I think it would be better, having a training. Also at school [undergraduate], in addition to what is there, there should be more ...." FGD participant ID 8*

> *"If we are updated [with training] it would be useful both for us and for them [psychiatry nurses] too. Since the load will decrease for them [psychiatry nurses] too." FGD participant ID 10*

> *"Yes and for the majority I think it is at that time [2014] that they were trained, I'm not sure if there were some training recently. But I would say that it needs to be updated every time." FGD participant ID 11*

Improving undergraduate psychiatry training and giving more attention to mental health aspects was also another suggestion given from the FGD participants.

> *"Why I supported number eight [FGD participant ID 8] is that if it can be linked with the study of the undergraduates... For example, if we work at ANC clinic there are tasks we perform here, right? things that are a must to do, things that you can't skip, right? Everyone knows that these are things they can perform, it is something that needs to be done. But this one [mental illness] we might be selective about it....There will be a mother that we might miss. So when we learn [in undergraduate] there must be a separate course that needs to be taken, that emphasizes that it is something we should do." FGD participant ID 5*

ANC assessment format doesn't have a place for mental health problems

A participant from the second FGD indicated that there was nothing that requires them to ask about psychological problems on their ANC assessment format and Health Management Information System (HMIS). They reported that this made them focus only on the things that were specified on the forms that they routinely use.

> *"We have formats, HMIS formats, starting from identification..... So in those, [mental health] can be included in some things. For example in ANC at HMIS there is her history about that... she has hepatitis B and C, RPR it includes such types. And it also includes HIV. But when it comes to psychology, psychiatric [conditions] where would it be put, if she was assessed? That should be improved and we will get used to it [assessing mental health]." FGD participant ID 11*

Involving Health Extension Workers (HEW)

Participants from both FGDs suggested training Health Extension Workers (HEWs) on maternal mental health problems. This was expected to improve depression detection because HEWs are close to women in the community and are positioned to be the primary contact for mothers. HEWs can also work on community awareness raising activities. Involving religious leaders in the awareness raising was also suggested.

> *"There is not much awareness [in the community], but if it is worked on the community there might be more cases that can be found because there are health extension workers [HEW]. They are the ones that are involved in that area and they are close with the mothers, and they will see them first before coming to us, they are also neighbors. So, more work should be done in that area. I think it is best if it is done there……Through them [HEW] you can get to the society since the extension workers are close to them and they work from house to house and they meet with them during meetings" FGD participant ID 1*

> *"When such kind of things occur [a mother develops depression] religious fathers in the holy water, they relate it [the illness] with other thing. When they [mothers] are depressed they would prefer to go to holy water place. So the community's perspective matters... they should all, like the midwives, be aware of this so that from the bottom we can have a uniform system" FGD participant ID 11*

4.5.4. Illness related influences

During the FGDs there were some discussions around the difficulty in differentiating normal emotional reaction from a depressive disorder. They also found it difficult because of the overlap between symptoms of depression and normal changes because of pregnancy; for example, fatigue. It was mentioned that PHC workers need to spend more time with people who have mental health problems in order to make the right diagnosis.

> *"It is difficult to differentiate depression as stated earlier. It might be part of the pregnancy. It can be a physiological change of pregnancy so it's difficult to differentiate. Identification might take a lot of time." FGD participant ID 8*

> *"For me it is easy to differentiate the psychotic ones but when it is depression, one mother can be depressed at some point and when she gets something to entertain her and when we counsel she might lighten up so I think that would be difficult to diagnose" FGD participant ID 3*

FGD participant ID 10: "As most of them indicated it is not thought to be easy [to identify depression]. Because to just assume right away that one person is not depressed, people may come just being bored. To identify if it is a real psychiatric case it needs proper counseling. So I don't think that's easy, it would be a challenge"

Interviewer: "It is a challenge. So what you are saying is it is not easy to differentiate those with symptoms from those whose symptoms are at the level of illness. But what makes it difficult?"

FGD participant ID 10: "At times people came here being just sad, because of different reasons. But to tell if it is depression or not... to know, it needs deep counseling. We need history, it may be family history, personal history. Just because that person is sad doesn't mean it is depression"

Chapter five: Discussion

When the study proposal was initially developed, the aim was to assess the referral and care pathways for pregnant women after a diagnosis of depression was made by primary care workers who had been trained in mhGAP through PRIME (Lund et al., 2012) in the Sodo district, rural Ethiopia. Before the start of data collection a half day refresher training on the mhGAP moderate to severe depression module was given to the ANC PHC workers, which was expected to improve detection. However, over a one month period there were no pregnant women diagnosed as having moderate to severe depression in the ANC clinics of the three health centres.

In the second month, we drew on the experience of the PRIME project (within which this study was nested), and introduced routine screening using a brief depression screening instrument (PHQ-9) in order to assist the PHC workers to identify cases. However, although there were pregnant women who scored above the validated cut-off on the PHQ-9 (5 and above), and this information was given to the primary care workers, still none of the primary care workers made a diagnosis of moderate to severe depression in the ANC clinics. This finding is in line with a Cochrane review, which concluded that use of depression screening or case finding instruments has little or no impact on detection of depression in primary care or general hospital (Gilbody et al., 2008). Because of the low/absent rates of detection of moderate to severe depression I was, therefore, unable to continue with the proposal as it was originally focused.

The current research project still focused on care pathways for pregnant women with moderate to severe depression, but at an earlier step in the care pathway - the detection of pregnant women with moderate to severe depression and challenges associated with identification of cases at a PHC level. The study tried to elaborate and understand factors which make this process challenging, both from the perspectives of women and health care providers. Finally I tried to come up with possible solutions for the identified problems together with the study subjects.

Participant recruitment for the first part of the current study, in-depth interviews with pregnant women with depression, was also a challenge because only a few women got a diagnosis of depression at the ANC clinics. Furthermore, pregnant women with a PHQ-9 score ≥5 (possible cases) tended not to attend the appointment date for interview or for reassessment by a research psychiatrist. Many of those who scored 5 and above on PHQ-9 and who showed up for reassessment were not diagnosed as having MDD. This can be explained in relation to the psychometric properties of the screening instrument used, i.e. low positive predictive value (PPV) at acceptable sensitivity, which made it difficult for routine use in clinical settings (Girma, 2013; Hanlon et al., 2015). Because of these challenges, I had to use a series of steps to recruit an adequate number of participants into the study. Details of participant recruitment steps can be found in the methods section under participant recruitment procedures.

From the study result, we can see that only three of the nine participants who scored high on PHQ-9 were diagnosed to have MDD by the research psychiatrist. Even though the majority did not have MDD, almost all had significant distressing emotional and physical symptom which made them a good candidate to study barriers to detection of common mental disorders (CMD) in the ANC clinics. The concept of CMD is broader than psychiatric diagnosis, referring to levels of depressive/anxiety symptoms considered to be clinically important, but not necessarily meeting diagnostic criteria (Goldberg, 1994). The concept of CMD has been found to be more culturally appropriate in the Ethiopian setting (Hanlon et al., 2008). Some of the participants who scored high on PHQ-9 were diagnosed by the research psychiatrist with anxiety disorder and somatic symptom disorder, rather than MDD, and this indicates the overlap between depression and other common mental disorder presentations (Goldberg, 2012).

5.1. Client level barriers

From the interviews with the women, a reluctance to disclose symptoms and seek help emerged as an important theme. This was explained as being due to a belief that there is little a PHC provider could do, the PHC provider not being the right person to talk to and fear of stigma and negative treatment by PHC worker. Disclosure of only physical symptoms during ANC consultation also appeared to be client level barrier to detection. The following client level barriers, which were in the conceptual framework we developed from literature, did not emerge during the IDIs with the women: mental health symptoms should not be disclosed at all, being able to cope without emotional help, embarrassment, hesitation to trouble the PHC provider and fear of loss of parental right.

As it can be seen from the findings of this current study, participating women were reluctant to discuss the non-somatic problems they had. They did not disclose emotional struggles they had to their ANC PHC worker. This finding is in keeping with findings from studies that have been conducted in many parts of the world (Cornford et al., 2007; Verhaak & Bensing, 2007; Yeung et al., 2004).The World Health Organization's mhGAP-IG includes a module on medically unexplained symptoms (WHO, 2016), which deserves greater attention to ensure that providers can recognize psychosomatic symptoms. However, it should not be assumed that all symptoms experienced by people who screen positive for depression are psychosomatic (Roberts et al., 2019).

Patients' explanatory model tells us how they make sense of a given episode of illness and how they choose and evaluate particular treatment (Kleinman, 1980). In order to understand why disclosure did not happen, it is very important to understand what symptoms the women had and what their explanatory model was, including what they thought might help with their symptoms.

All participating women had both physical and non-physical symptoms which were distressing to them. The mixture of symptoms they reported on PHQ-9 and the PHQ scores above the validated threshold in this setting supports that (Kroenke & Spitzer, 2002).

If the women had symptoms, why were those not communicated? Here, I will focus on factors from the women side. Provider, illness and system level factors will be discussed separately. This will again lead to the question of whether women perceived the symptoms they had as a problem or not. I would argue that most women saw their symptoms as problematic, because these symptoms were reported by the pregnant women during the in-depth interviews when they were asked to report what problems they had.

The kind of problem women thought they had differed depending on the explanatory model they used. Some considered symptoms as a medical problem (physical problem or mental health problem). Others thought of symptoms as caused by supernatural forces like bad spirit, Satan, bewitchment or punishment from God because of family's wrong doing. For others, it was a consequence of economic hardship, marital difficulty or other life stressors. Other studies have shown that it is very common to attribute mental illness to psychosocial stressors and supernatural causes (Mayston et al., 2019; Mulatu, 1999; Roberts et al., 2019). Most women had more than one explanatory model for the symptoms they had. Indeed, the majority of women mentioned multiple different factors that had contributed to development of symptoms. This finding is supported by the biopsychosocial model of depression which emphasizes on the importance of considering both biological and psychosocial variables in depression (Ross, Sellers, Gilbert Evans, & Romach, 2004).

Understanding whether or not women wanted help for the symptoms or problems they had is also very important. Most women wanted help, but the kind of things they thought might help differed and was somehow related to what they thought the cause was. For those with non-medical explanations, the health centre or hospital was not seen as a place to seek help. For these women, prayer, holy water and traditional treatments were preferred. For those with significant financial or relationship difficulties, resolution of those difficulties was thought to help improve symptoms. A study on depressed postpartum women from Ethiopia showed that even though the majority of women reported that they needed professional help for their symptoms, many women relied on non-professional sources of help such as from their partner, parents and friends. Equal proportions of women endorsed biomedical health care and traditional or religious healing (Azale et al., 2016).

Even for women with medical explanations, disclosure of symptoms to ANC PHC workers was affected by the type of illness they suspected they had. For problems related to the pregnancy and the fetus, ANC clinic was seen as the best place. For mental illness, psychiatric clinics were thought to be appropriate. In the study site, even if symptoms are recognized as a manifestation of mental illness, non-modern treatment settings are more acceptable. An old study from Ethiopia showed that traditional treatment methods were preferred more often for treating symptoms of mental disorders and modern medicine was preferred more often for treating physical diseases or symptoms (Alem, Jacobsson, Araya, Kebede, & Kullgren, 1999; Mulatu, 1999). Recent studies show that biomedical treatments are becoming more acceptable in perinatal population (Azale et al., 2016).

There is convincing evidence regarding the role of stressful life events, social conflict and food insecurity and hunger in determining depression (Patel et al., 2010). Poverty is consistently associated with increased prevalence of adult CMD, such as depression and anxiety disorders globally and the effects of poverty on mental illness are more pronounced among women particularly during the perinatal period (Lund et al., 2018). Our participating women had multiple problems - medical, marital, financial - and their needs included alleviation of marital conflict and a route out of poverty. This phenomenon has been well described in a study from rural India which showed patients' need included greater economic security, better working conditions, accountability and quality improvements in the public health system, reduced family conflict, and a route out of poverty for their children (Roberts et al., 2019). Primary care is unlikely to be the best platform to address those needs, although primary care workers may have a role in identifying and referring individuals in need of such support. In a context where many illness related problems are associated with poverty, initiatives which fall outside the strict boundaries of health care are required. In their absence, health care providers working in these contexts cannot be expected to provide a comprehensive care (Petersen, 2000).

5.2. Provider level barriers

The interview and FGD data showed provider level barriers to the diagnosis of depression in the ANC clinics included low confidence, low skill, poor therapeutic alliance, short consultation time, not exploring further when faced with diagnostic difficulties, low index of suspicion, rare inquiry about depressive symptoms, distraction by other presenting problems and reluctance to label patients as depressed. As a whole, lack of experience, short practice time of PHC workers, lack of interest in mental health and lack of willingness to look for signs of depression did not emerge as provider level barriers to diagnosing depression in ANC clinics.

A major provider factor that appeared to influence detection is how the clinician interviews the patient (Goldberg et al., 1993). Asking about depressive symptoms during consultation leads to a diagnosis of depression and some form of depression treatment. This might be one factor that can explain the low rates of detection of depression in our ANC clinics as 'not asking about depressive symptoms' was a recurrent theme both in the in-depth interviews and FGDs. Most clients were willing to report psychological symptoms they had if they had been asked, which again was similar with findings in the literature (Simon, VonKorff, Piccinelli, Fullerton, & Ormel, 1999; Williams Jr et al., 1999). Their willingness was implied, in addition to their words, from the fact that they readily reported symptoms while being interviewed by data collectors on PHQ-9 and during the in-depth interviews.

There was a conflict between what women and some ANC PHC workers were saying regarding disclosure of symptoms. The women were willing to report symptoms during ANC consultations if asked, even though they did not necessarily see ANC PHC workers as the best people to help them, but they were not encouraged and given the space to do so; while rural ANC PHC workers thought that women would share their symptoms if they had any without the need to probe or opening up the space for them to report. This indicates PHC workers' lack of awareness and, not paying attention to the sensitive nature of the problem and the need for good relationship and trust for disclosure of psychiatric symptoms. Unlike findings from a HIC (Chew-Graham, Sharp, Chamberlain, Folkes, & Turner, 2009), ANC PHC workers in this setting did not seem to make conscious decisions in their everyday work about whether to facilitate women's disclosure of symptoms of depression.

The way that assessment questions were phrased was also a contributing factor for lack of detection of depression in the ANC clinics. Communication strategies that predict successful recognition of depression are the use of broad, open ended psychosocial questions and a proportion of the interview devoted to emotional problems (Carney et al., 1999). This was not practiced in the study site health centres as evidenced by discussions during the FGDs. The 'Health systems strengthening in sub-Saharan Africa' (ASSET) research project in Ethiopia is trying to address this problem through training health workers in clinical communication skills

(Feyissa et al., 2019). This emphasis on clinical communication skills is also in support of the health sector transformation plan agenda of the Ministry of Health of Ethiopia to promote compassionate, respectful clinicians (FMoH, 2015).

There was reluctance, by the ANC PHC workers, to label women as depressed. This seems to be similar in the other PHC clinics as well, as PHC workers, when asked why diagnosis of depression was very low, they said that it was worse to give their patients a label of depression and better just to treat them symptomatically[1]. This might be linked to the stigma of mental illness. The added dimension in the current study is pregnancy. Perhaps any illness evokes fear in the woman, regardless of whether mental or physical. According to (Hanlon et al., 2010), pregnant women were worried about surviving pregnancy, so perhaps anything that seems like a problem in pregnancy will be very worrying for them.

5.3. System level barriers

There are multiple challenges to provision of maternal mental health care in LMICs. A situational analysis from five LMICs, including Ethiopia, identified one challenge to be the limited evidence on feasible detection and treatment strategies for maternal mental disorders (Baron et al., 2016). From the conceptual framework presented in the literature review (see Figure 1), workload, lack of time and inadequate training (insufficient undergraduate training on mental health and insufficient on the job training) emerged from the FGDs as system level barriers for diagnosis of depression in the ANC clinics. Lack of access to mental health specialist and lack of appropriate referral pathways were not supported by our participants as all ANC PHC workers mentioned that they can easily refer cases to a psychiatric nurse or to a mental health focal person. Other potential system level barriers for identification of depression in PHC - poor reimbursement for depression treatment, lack of accessible assessment tool for depression and lack of resources like proper psychosocial interventions - did not emerge in any of the FGDs.

---

[1]After the PRIME research project trained the Sodo district PHC workers on mhGAP-IG, they were not detecting as many depression cases as expected. A member of the research team met with the PHC workers and tried to understand why that was. They said, among other things, for depressionit was worse to give the woman a label of a mental illness and was better to just treat them symptomatically (personal communication).

One reason raised for not routinely doing a mental health assessment was because it was not part of the ANC assessment form that ANC PHC workers use during clinical consultations. Similarly, maternal mental health care indicators were not part of the health management information system (HMIS). Because of this, PHC workers are more likely to focus on the mandatory assessments mentioned in the evaluation format they use, like screening for infections and focusing on obstetric care. The Perinatal Mental Health Project in South Africa (Honikman et al., 2004) showed that maternity health workers may be trained to screen and refer for mental distress in low-resource primary care settings but for it to be successful; presence of on-going supervision and support, established protocol and referral systems, consistency with offering screening and involvement of clinical coordinator are very important (Honikman, Van Heyningen, Field, Baron, & Tomlinson, 2012).

Routine use of depression screening instrument in the ANC clinics, to better identify those with clinical depression, may not, however, be the best solution because of a number of reasons. First, cross-sectional screening might detect large numbers of false positives because of the transient nature of mood changes in many people (Gilbody et al., 2006). As an example, two of our IDI participants (ID 101 and 302) fulfilled diagnostic criteria for MDD at the time of screening but when assessed by the research psychiatrist at the time of the interview, were doing well, as their social problems had largely resolved since the screening. Evidence-based treatment guidelines recommend an initial period of watchful waiting before active intervention for mild to moderate depression and many missed cases that will benefit from treatment will be identified during later visits, so screening may not be efficient (Gilbody et al., 2006). Second, the low prevalence (3.9%) of depression in ANC clinics (Girma, 2013) means that even sensitive and specific instruments will have low positive predictive value (PPV) (Girma, 2013; Hanlon et al., 2015). Low PPV will make the test less useful for clinicians, because patients will be followed up unnecessarily. Third, according to Gilbody and colleagues (2006) "identifying a large number of patients with depression could divert resources from patients with greater need, who would benefit more. Screening also increases the length of time needed for consultation in primary care, when follow-up interviews and further diagnostic investigations are required."

In Ethiopia, only 'behavioral disorders' and 'epilepsy' are collected as mental health indicators from routine HMIS at a primary care level. No information can be found on coverage of maternal mental health care in Ethiopia as the HMIS does not contain indicators for maternal mental ill-health (Baron et al., 2016). Due to competing priorities, the HMIS appears to be more geared to communicable diseases, overlooking the need for information on non-communicable diseases. The insufficiency of mental health indicators in existing HMIS has been recognized in other LMICs as well and efforts to include additional indicators are being made (Upadhaya et al., 2016). The 'Emerging mental health systems in low and middle income countries' (Emerald) research programme, which aimed to support mental health systems strengthening in the six countries, including Ethiopia, introduced, implemented and evaluated new procedures for collecting mental health indicators and, overall, the new indicators were found to be feasible in the primary care facilities (Ahuja et al., 2019).

Another reason for lower detection of depression raised by PHC workers is the fact that a woman will not be followed by the same PHC provider every time she comes for follow up. FGD participants from ANC clinics mentioned that women prefer to be seen by the same ANC PHC worker every time they come and that would have helped in the establishment of a relationship and trust. The amount of contact a provider has with the patient has been established as an important predictor of detection in primary care (Mitchell, 2010). This problem is not unique to the ANC setting as research in other clinics in Ethiopia also showed that patients are rarely seen more than once and that clinicians and patients rarely form ongoing therapeutic relations. This was noted as one reason for the low detection of depression at PHC level (Fekadu et al., 2017).

Lack of time and high work load is a barrier to adequate attention being given to depression in PHC (Hirschfeld et al., 1997; Mitchell, 2010). This was raised as a major problem during FGDs with ANC PHC workers from urban sites, and participants mentioned the details of how it has affected their practice. Yet, this is not a universal finding as in many of the rural clinics, the workload was not as high, as described by the women and ANC PHC workers. The women reported that they felt that they would be able to talk to ANC PHC workers if they had thought discussing their problem was appropriate. This is a very positive finding and will give a good opportunity to integrate mental health care with maternal health services.

The low level of knowledge and skill of PHC clinicians will have an important impact on diagnosis of depression (Fekadu et al., 2017). Inadequate undergraduate and on-the-job training is one factor affecting the knowledge, skill and confidence of PHC workers to identify and care for patients with depression (Hirschfeld et al., 1997; Mitchell, 2010). FGD participants acknowledged the gap in undergraduate as well as on-the-job training. Training PHC workers on maternal mental health conditions can contribute to addressing this problem.

Raising awareness in the community is also very important. Health extension workers (HEWs) are widely used in Ethiopia to provide care for a broad range of health issues. They have contributed substantially to the improvement in women's utilization of family planning, antenatal care and HIV testing (Medhanyie et al., 2012). In the same way, HEWs can be used to increase awareness in the community and improve women's access to mental health care in ANC clinics by referring depressed women to midwives at health centres. As traditional treatment settings are often preferred for treating symptoms of mental disorders in Ethiopia (Alem et al., 1999), raising awareness of traditional healers and religious leaders on depression would be very important. They will be able to refer women with severe symptoms who might benefit from medical treatment.

5.4. Illness related influences

From the conceptual framework developed in Chapter 2, difficulty in differentiating normal emotional reactions from that of depression and overlap between symptoms of pregnancy and symptoms of depression emerged from the FGDs as illness related influences in identifying depression in the ANC clinics. Things listed under illness complexity (mental illness is difficult to deal with and awkward to diagnose, somatic complaints which are thought to have psychological bases are perceived as difficult) and presence of comorbidity, which might create ambiguity and diagnostic difficulties, did not emerge during the discussions we had with ANC PHC workers.

Determining the boundary between a clinical disorder and subclinical symptoms is complex, and non-mental health workers report difficulty distinguishing between distress caused by significant life stressors and psychiatric illness like depression (Johnston et al., 2007). Higher severity of depression is associated with greater recognition in PHC (Naqvi & Khan, 2005). A study from rural Ethiopia showed that depression cases identified by PHC clinicians were those with high symptom burden, suicidality and functional impairment (Habtamu et al., 2019). Because of the very low rate of detection of depression in the study site ANC clinics, we think in addition to milder forms also those with severe illnesses, who are more likely to benefit from treatment, are left undetected (Fekadu et al., 2017). Thus this illness related influence might not fully explain the low rates of detection of depression in the ANC clinics.

It is expected that women will experience physiological changes during pregnancy and physical symptoms like change in energy level, sleep and appetite, which can overlap with symptoms of depression (Matthey & Ross-Hamid, 2011). A difficulty faced when measuring depression in the perinatal period is that somatic symptoms related to pregnancy might be mistakenly attributed to the depressive syndrome. In the current study, almost all women were able to differentiate and comment on normal pregnancy changes from the symptoms they described as problems by comparing their current pregnancy with the previous one. A study from Malawi showed that the psychological subscale of Self Reporting Questionnaire (SRQ), which excluded all somatic symptoms from screening scale, was not significantly different from that of the total SRQ, indicating that the inclusion of the somatic items did not affect the test performance of the instrument (Stewart et al., 2009). In a study from Ethiopia, the number of somatic symptoms was strongly correlated with emotional symptoms during pregnancy and somatic symptoms were independently associated with worse maternal functional impairment (Senturk et al., 2012). Again, in a population-based study, complaints of fatigue were associated strongly with maternal CMD but not with the presence of physical ill-health, anemia or under-nutrition (Smartt et al., 2016). Thus, any report of significant somatic compliant by pregnant women should not be taken lightly as it may be a potential indicator of CMD.

Limitations

The qualitative design was well suited to addressing the research question of this study as the aim was to gain a deep understanding of the process of detection of depression in the ANC clinics including the experiences of women and care providers.

As the design was qualitative, it has the drawback of not being able to verify the result objectively and not being generalizable. In addition, the current study has the following limitations.

- Interviewer bias: I, as a psychiatrist, have my own understanding of depression and other CMDs. There is always a risk of unconsciously influencing the response of participants. I have tried to reduce introducing my bias by being conscious of this phenomenon during discussion with the women.
- During the in-depth interviews, women were spontaneously reporting non-physical/emotional symptoms as a problem. This was not practiced in their regular follow ups with PHC workers. This reporting could have been influenced by the administration of PHQ-9 to participants in the weeks before the interview and being linked to a mental health focal person or psychiatric nurse before they were interviewed by the researcher. Their explanatory model might have been affected due to this encounter.
- The data collector during IDIs and FGDs was a psychiatrist and participants were aware of that. In addition, the researcher was involved in mhGAP training of PHC workers and is familiar to many of the ANC PHC workers. This potentially has introduced social desirability bias
- The current study did not gather information from all important stakeholders like family, HEWs and health institution management as understanding their perspective is an important factor in designing interventions for the problems identified.
- The number of pregnant women screened with PHQ-9 by data collectors and ANC PHC workers was not documented as this was not required by the research question. The screening of pregnant women was not part of a larger study either.

Conclusion and Recommendations

Although detection of depression does not equate to good clinical care, it is the first critical step in the process (Miller, Shade, & Vasireddy, 2009). Multiple patient, provider and system-level barriers to detection of depression in pregnant women in ANC clinics of health centres and primary hospital were identified in the current study. PHC workers included in the study suggested asking depression specific questions during follow-ups, giving more time to women who have mental health problems, ensuring mothers privacy and maintaining confidentiality by improving the ANC clinic setting, arranging all ANC follow ups with the same PHC worker, including mental health assessment in the ANC assessment format and HMIS, and training HEWs on maternal mental health and raising awareness of religious leaders and the community, as a solution to improve the detection of depression in their clinics. In addition, they gave strong emphasis to the need for improving undergraduate psychiatry training, regular on-the-job mental health training, follow up and supervision, and sharing experience from those who have better expertise as a way of improving their depression assessment skills.

The identified barriers, and the suggested approaches to overcome the barriers, call for interventions at different levels; awareness-raising at a community level, training on mental disorders and clinical communication skills at a provider level and enabling the health care system to support the integration of mental health care into maternal health services at a higher level. This can be achieved by making the environment suitable for mental health assessment and treatment; e.g. having individual consultation rooms available, revising the undergraduate training curriculum to include mental health care, providing regular and updated on-the-job training courses with regular follow-up, monitoring, support and supervision and making mental health assessment part of the routine ANC service, by including it as part of the assessment format and HMIS.

According to the 'Improving Detection of Depression in Primary care in Sub-Saharan Africa' (IDEAS) study, "in order to achieve improved detection, the first crucial step is to understand what the manifestations and presentations of depression are in the local context. The second step is to understand the factors that may affect detection, for example how the health system and health facilities are set up, how the actual clinical encounter is facilitated, the attitudes and expectations of provider and receiver, and the broader social context." Follow-up studies are thus required to better understand the experiences of women and providers, to quantify the magnitude of the problem and to develop and evaluate contextually appropriate interventions to improve the detection of depression in pregnant women.

References

Alem, A., Jacobsson, L., Araya, M., Kebede, D., & Kullgren, G. (1999). How are mental disorders seen and where is help sought in a rural Ethiopian community? A key informant study in Butajira, Ethiopia. *Acta Psychiatrica Scandinavica, 100*, 40-47.

Alem, A., Kebede, D., Fekadu, A., Shibre, T., Fekadu, D., Beyero, T., . . . Kullgren, G. (2009). Clinical course and outcome of schizophrenia in a predominantly treatment-naive cohort in rural Ethiopia. *Schizophrenia bulletin, 35*(3), 646-654.

Ali, G.-C., Ryan, G., & De Silva, M. J. (2016). Validated screening tools for common mental disorders in low and middle income countries: a systematic review. *PLoS One, 11*(6), e0156939.

Ayano, G., Tesfaw, G., & Shumet, S. (2019). Prevalence and determinants of antenatal depression in Ethiopia: A systematic review and meta-analysis. *PLoS One, 14*(2), e0211764.

Ayinde, O. O., Oladeji, B. D., Abdulmalik, J., Jordan, K., Kola, L., & Gureje, O. (2018). Quality of perinatal depression care in primary care setting in Nigeria. *BMC Health Serv Res, 18*(1), 879. doi: 10.1186/s12913-018-3716-3

Azale, T., Fekadu, A., & Hanlon, C. (2016). Treatment gap and help-seeking for postpartum depression in a rural African setting. *BMC Psychiatry, 16*(1), 196.

Barkow, K., Heun, R., Üstün, T. B., Berger, M., Bermejo, I., Gaebel, W., . . . Maier, W. (2004). Identification of somatic and anxiety symptoms which contribute to the detection of depression in primary health care. *European Psychiatry, 19*(5), 250-257.

Baron, E. C., Hanlon, C., Mall, S., Honikman, S., Breuer, E., Kathree, T., . . . Tomlinson, M. (2016). Maternal mental health in primary care in five low- and middle-income countries: a situational analysis. *BMC Health Serv Res, 16*, 53. doi: 10.1186/s12913-016-1291-z

Byatt, N., Biebel, K., Friedman, L., Debordes-Jackson, G., Ziedonis, D., & Pbert, L. (2013). Patient's views on depression care in obstetric settings: how do they compare to the views of perinatal health care professionals? *Gen Hosp Psychiatry, 35*(6), 598-604.

Byatt, N., Biebel, K., Lundquist, R. S., Moore Simas, T. A., Debordes-Jackson, G., Allison, J., & Ziedonis, D. (2012). Patient, provider, and system-level barriers and facilitators to addressing perinatal depression. *Journal of Reproductive and Infant Psychology, 30*(5), 436-449.

Cape, J., & McCulloch, Y. (1999). Patients' reasons for not presenting emotional problems in general practice consultations. *Br J Gen Pract, 49*(448), 875-879.

Carney, P. A., Eliassen, M. S., Wolford, G. L., Owen, M., Badger, L. W., & Dietrich, A. J. (1999). How physician communication influences recognition of depression in primary care. *Journal of Family Practice, 48*(12), 958-958.

Carson, A., Stone, J., Warlow, C., & Sharpe, M. (2004). Patients whom neurologists find difficult to help. *Journal of Neurology, Neurosurgery & Psychiatry, 75*(12), 1776-1778.

Chew-Graham, C. A., Sharp, D., Chamberlain, E., Folkes, L., & Turner, K. M. (2009). Disclosure of symptoms of postnatal depression, the perspectives of health professionals and women: a qualitative study. *BMC family practice, 10*(1), 7.

Cornford, C. S., Hill, A., & Reilly, J. (2007). How patients with depressive symptoms view their condition: a qualitative study. *Family Practice, 24*(4), 358-364.

Coyne, J. C., Klinkman, M. S., Gallo, S. M., & Schwenk, T. L. (1997). Short-term outcomes of detected and undetected depressed primary care patients and depressed psychiatric patients. *Gen Hosp Psychiatry, 19*(5), 333-343.

Cuijpers, P., van Straten, A., van Schaik, A., & Andersson, G. (2009). Psychological treatment of depression in primary care: a meta-analysis. *British journal of general practice, 59*(559), e51-e60.

Del Piccolo, L., Saltini, A., Zimmermann, C., & Dunn, G. (2000). Differences in verbal behaviours of patients with and without emotional distress during primary care consultations. *Psychol Med, 30*(3), 629-643.

Deveugele, M., Derese, A., & De Maeseneer, J. (2002). Is GP–patient communication related to their perceptions of illness severity, coping and social support? *Social science & medicine, 55*(7), 1245-1253.

Fekadu, A., Demissie, M., Birhane, R., Medhin, G., Bitew, T., Hailemariam, M., . . . Petersen, I. (2020). Under detection of depression in primary care settings in low and middle-income countries: A systematic review and meta-analysis. *medRxiv*.

Fekadu, A., Hanlon, C., Medhin, G., Alem, A., Selamu, M., Giorgis, T. W., . . . Breuer, E. (2016). Development of a scalable mental healthcare plan for a rural district in Ethiopia. *The British Journal of Psychiatry, 208*(s56), s4-s12.

Fekadu, A., Medhin, G., Selamu, M., Giorgis, T. W., Lund, C., Alem, A., . . . Hanlon, C. (2017). Recognition of depression by primary care clinicians in rural Ethiopia. *Contemp Clin Trials, 18*(1), 56. doi: 10.1016/j.cct.2017.06.013

Feyissa, Y. M., Hanlon, C., Emyu, S., Cornick, R. V., Fairall, L., Gebremichael, D., . . . Mamo, Y. (2019). Using a mentorship model to localise the Practical Approach to Care Kit (PACK): from South Africa to Ethiopia. *BMJ global health, 3*(Suppl 5), e001108.

Fisher, J., Cabral de Mello, M., Patel, V., Rahman, A., Tran, T., Holton, S., & Holmes, W. (2012). Prevalence and determinants of common perinatal mental disorders in women in low- and lower-middle-income countries: a systematic review. *Bull World Health Organ, 90*(2), 139g-149g. doi: 10.2471/blt.11.091850

Floyd, B. J. (1997). Problems in accurate medical diagnosis of depression in female patients. Social science & medicine, 44(3), 403-412.

FMoH, E. (2015). Health Sector Transformation Plan: HSTP 2015/16-2019/20. August.

Fonseca, A., Gorayeb, R., & Canavarro, M. C. (2015). Women' s help-seeking behaviours for depressive symptoms during the perinatal period: Socio-demographic and clinical correlates and perceived barriers to seeking professional help. *Midwifery, 31*(12), 1177-1185.

Gale, N. K., Heath, G., Cameron, E., Rashid, S., & Redwood, S. (2013). Using the framework method for the analysis of qualitative data in multi-disciplinary health research. *BMC medical research methodology, 13*(1), 1-8.

Gelaye, B., Rondon, M. B., Araya, R., & Williams, M. A. (2016). Epidemiology of maternal depression, risk factors, and child outcomes in low-income and middle-income countries. *The Lancet Psychiatry, 3*(10), 973-982.

Gelaye, B., Williams, M. A., Lemma, S., Deyessa, N., Bahretibeb, Y., Shibre, T., . . . Vander Stoep, A. (2013). Validity of the patient health questionnaire-9 for depression screening and diagnosis in East Africa. *Psychiatry research, 210*(2), 653-661.

Gilbody, S., Sheldon, T., & House, A. (2008). Screening and case-finding instruments for depression: a meta-analysis. *Cmaj, 178*(8), 997-1003.

Gilbody, S., Sheldon, T., & Wessely, S. (2006). Should we screen for depression? *Bmj, 332*(7548), 1027-1030.

Girma, F., Hanlon, C. (2013). Detecting depression during pregnancy: validation of PHQ-9, Kessler-10, Kessler-6 and SRQ-20 in Butajira area health centres antenatal care clinics, Ethiopia. A book for a post-graduate degree (certificate in psychiatry). Unpublished

Glover, V., O'Donnell, K. J., O'Connor, T. G., & Fisher, J. (2018). Prenatal maternal stress, fetal programming, and mechanisms underlying later psychopathology—A global perspective. *Development and Psychopathology, 30*(3), 843-854.

Goldberg, D. (1994). A bio-social model for common mental disorders. *Acta Psychiatrica Scandinavica, 90*, 66-70.

Goldberg, D. (2012). The overlap between the common mental disorders–Challenges for classification. *International Review Of Psychiatry, 24*(6), 549-555.

Goldberg, D. P., Jenkins, L., Millar, T., & Faragher, E. (1993). The ability of trainee general practitioners to identify psychological distress among their patients. *Psychol Med, 23*(1), 185-193.

Grigoriadis, S., VonderPorten, E. H., Mamisashvili, L., Tomlinson, G., Dennis, C.-L., Koren, G., . . . Radford, K. (2013). The impact of maternal depression during pregnancy on perinatal outcomes: a systematic review and meta-analysis. *The Journal of clinical psychiatry, 74*(4), e321-341.

Habtamu, K., Medhin, G., Selamu, M., Tirfessa, K., Hanlon, C., & Fekadu, A. (2019). Functional impairment among people diagnosed with depression in primary healthcare in rural Ethiopia: a comparative cross-sectional study. *Int J Ment Health Syst, 13*(1), 50.

Hahn, S. R. (2001). Physical symptoms and physician-experienced difficulty in the physician–patient relationship. *Annals of internal medicine, 134*(9_Part_2), 897-904.

Hailemariam, M., Fekadu, A., Medhin, G., Prince, M., & Hanlon, C. (2019). Equitable access to mental healthcare integrated in primary care for people with severe mental disorders in rural Ethiopia: a community-based cross-sectional study. Int J Ment Health Syst, 13(1), 1-10.

Hanlon, C., Medhin, G., Alem, A., Araya, M., Abdulahi, A., Tesfaye, M., . . . Baheretibeb, Y. (2008). Measuring common mental disorders in women in Ethiopia. *Soc Psychiatry Psychiatr Epidemiol, 43*(8), 653.

Hanlon, C., Medhin, G., Alem, A., Tesfaye, F., Lakew, Z., Worku, B., . . . Hughes, M. (2009). Impact of antenatal common mental disorders upon perinatal outcomes in Ethiopia: the P-MaMiE population-based cohort study. *Tropical Medicine & International Health, 14*(2), 156-166.

Hanlon, C., Medhin, G., Selamu, M., Birhane, R., Dewey, M., Tirfessa, K., . . . Patel, V. (2020). Impact of integrated district level mental health care on clinical and social outcomes of people with severe mental illness in rural Ethiopia: an intervention cohort study. Epidemiology and psychiatric sciences, 29.

Hanlon, C., Medhin, G., Selamu, M., Breuer, E., Worku, B., Hailemariam, M., . . . Fekadu, A. (2015). Validity of brief screening questionnaires to detect depression in primary care in Ethiopia. *J Affect Disord, 186*, 32-39.

Hanlon, C., Whitley, R., Wondimagegn, D., Alem, A., & Prince, M. (2010). Between life and death: exploring the sociocultural context of antenatal mental distress in rural Ethiopia. *Arch Womens Ment Health, 13*(5), 385-393.

Hirschfeld, R. M., Keller, M. B., Panico, S., Arons, B. S., Barlow, D., Davidoff, F., . . . Gorman, J. M. (1997). The National Depressive and Manic-Depressive Association consensus statement on the undertreatment of depression. *Jama, 277*(4), 333-340.

Honikman, S., Rosenthal, H., Faure, S., Wirz, B., van Zijl, S., Littlejohn, M., & Bergman, N. (2004). The Perinatal Mental Health Project. *Mental Health Promotion Case Studies from Countries, 38*, 82.

Honikman, S., Van Heyningen, T., Field, S., Baron, E., & Tomlinson, M. (2012). Stepped care for maternal mental health: a case study of the perinatal mental health project in South Africa. *PLoS Med, 9*(5).

Ishikawa, H., Takayama, T., Yamazaki, Y., Seki, Y., Katsumata, N., & Aoki, Y. (2002). The interaction between physician and patient communication behaviors in Japanese cancer consultations and the influence of personal and consultation characteristics. *Patient education and counseling, 46*(4), 277-285.

Jenkins, R., Othieno, C., Okeyo, S., Kaseje, D., Aruwa, J., Oyugi, H., . . . Kauye, F. (2013). Short structured general mental health in service training programme in Kenya improves patient health and social outcomes but not detection of mental health problems-a pragmatic cluster randomised controlled trial. *Int J Ment Health Syst, 7*(1), 25.

Johnston, O., Kumar, S., Kendall, K., Peveler, R., Gabbay, J., & Kendrick, T. (2007). Qualitative study of depression management in primary care: GP and patient goals, and the value of listening. *Br J Gen Pract, 57*(544), e1-e14.

Jordans, M. J. D., & Luitel, N. P. (2019). Community-, facility-, and individual-level outcomes of a district mental healthcare plan in a low-resource setting in Nepal: A population-based evaluation. *16*(2), e1002748. doi: 10.1371/journal.pmed.1002748

Kauye, F., Jenkins, R., & Rahman, A. (2014). Training primary health care workers in mental health and its impact on diagnoses of common mental disorders in primary care of a developing country, Malawi: a cluster-randomized controlled trial. *Psychol Med, 44*(3), 657-666. Kleinman, A. (1980). *Patients and healers in the context of culture: An exploration of the borderland between anthropology, medicine, and psychiatry* (Vol. 3): Univ of California Press.

Kohn, R., Saxena, S., Levav, I., & Saraceno, B. (2004). The treatment gap in mental health care. *Bull World Health Organ, 82*, 858-866.

Kohrt, B. A., Jordans, M. J., Turner, E. L., Sikkema, K. J., Luitel, N. P., Rai, S., . . . Patel, V. (2018). Reducing stigma among healthcare providers to improve mental health services (RESHAPE): protocol for a pilot cluster randomized controlled trial of a stigma reduction intervention for training primary healthcare workers in Nepal. *Pilot and feasibility studies, 4*(1), 36.

Kroenke, K., & Spitzer, R. L. (2002). The PHQ-9: a new depression diagnostic and severity measure. *Psychiatric annals, 32*(9), 509-515.

Kroenke, K., Spitzer, R. L., & Williams, J. B. (2001). The Phq-9. *Journal of general internal medicine, 16*(9), 606-613.

Luitel, N. P. (2017). Treatment gap and barriers for mental health care: A cross-sectional community survey in Nepal. *Int J Ment Health Syst, 12*(8), e0183223. doi: 10.1186/s13033-017-0169-8

Lund, C., Brooke-Sumner, C., Baingana, F., Baron, E. C., Breuer, E., Chandra, P., . . . Kieling, C. (2018). Social determinants of mental disorders and the Sustainable Development Goals: a systematic review of reviews. *The Lancet Psychiatry, 5*(4), 357-369.

Lund, C., Tomlinson, M., De Silva, M., Fekadu, A., Shidhaye, R., Jordans, M., . . . Prince, M. (2012). PRIME: a programme to reduce the treatment gap for mental disorders in five low-and middle-income countries. *PLoS medicine, 9*(12), e1001359.

Maguire, P. (2002). Improving the recognition of concerns and affective disorders in cancer patients. *Annals of oncology, 13*(suppl_4), 177-181.

Matthey, S., & Ross-Hamid, C. (2011). The validity of DSM symptoms for depression and anxiety disorders during pregnancy. *J Affect Disord, 133*(3), 546-552.

Mayston, R., Frissa, S., Tekola, B., Hanlon, C., Prince, M., & Fekadu, A. (2019). Explanatory models of depression in sub-Saharan Africa: Synthesis of qualitative evidence. *Social science & medicine*, 112760.

McConley, R. L., Mrug, S., Gilliland, M. J., Lowry, R., Elliott, M. N., Schuster, M. A., . . . Franklin, F. A. (2011). Mediators of maternal depression and family structure on child BMI: parenting quality and risk factors for child overweight. *Obesity, 19*(2), 345-352.

Medhanyie, A., Spigt, M., Kifle, Y., Schaay, N., Sanders, D., Blanco, R., . . . Berhane, Y. (2012). The role of health extension workers in improving utilization of maternal health services in rural areas in Ethiopia: a cross sectional study. *BMC Health Serv Res, 12*(1), 352.

Mersha, A. G., Abebe, S. A., Sori, L. M., & Abegaz, T. M. (2018). Prevalence and associated factors of perinatal depression in Ethiopia: a systematic review and meta-analysis. *Depress Res Treat, 2018*.

Milgrom, J., & Gemmill, A. W. (2014). Screening for perinatal depression. *Best Practice & Research Clinical Obstetrics & Gynaecology, 28*(1), 13-23.

Miller, L., Shade, M., & Vasireddy, V. (2009). Beyond screening: assessment of perinatal depression in a perinatal care setting. *Arch Womens Ment Health, 12*(5), 329.

Mitchell, A. J. (2010). Why do clinicians have difficulty detecting depression. *Screening for depression in clinical practice: An evidence-based guide*, 57-82.

Mitchell, A. J., Vaze, A., & Rao, S. (2009). Clinical diagnosis of depression in primary care: a meta-analysis. *The Lancet, 374*(9690), 609-619.

Mulatu, M. S. (1999). Perceptions of mental and physical illnesses in north-western Ethiopia: causes, treatments, and attitudes. *Journal of health psychology, 4*(4), 531-549.

Naqvi, H., & Khan, M. M. (2005). Depression in primary care: difficulties and paradoxes. *J Pak Med Assoc, 55*(9), 393-398.

Nease, D. E., Klinkman, M. S., & Volk, R. J. (2002). Improved detection of depression in primary care through severity evaluation. *Journal of Family Practice, 51*(12), 1065-1071.

Noonan, M., Doody, O., Jomeen, J., & Galvin, R. (2017). Midwives' perceptions and experiences of caring for women who experience perinatal mental health problems: an integrative review. *Midwifery, 45*, 56-71.

Padmanathan, P., & De Silva, M. J. (2013). The acceptability and feasibility of task-sharing for mental healthcare in low and middle income countries: a systematic review. *Social science & medicine, 97*, 82-86.

Patel, V. (1996). Recognition of common mental disorders in primary care in African countries: should" mental" be dropped? *The Lancet, 347*(9003), 742-744.

Patel, V., Lund, C., Hatherill, S., Plagerson, S., Corrigall, J., Funk, M., & Flisher, A. J. (2010). Mental disorders: equity and social determinants. *Equity, social determinants and public health programmes, 115*, 134.

Patel, V., & Prince, M. (2006). Maternal psychological morbidity and low birth weight in India. *The British Journal of Psychiatry, 188*(3), 284-285.

Patel, V., Rodrigues, M., & DeSouza, N. (2002). Gender, poverty, and postnatal depression: a study of mothers in Goa, India. *American journal of Psychiatry, 159*(1), 43-47.

Patel, V., Simon, G., Chowdhary, N., Kaaya, S., & Araya, R. (2009). Packages of care for depression in low- and middle-income countries. *PLoS Med, 6*(10), e1000159.

Petersen, I. (2000). Comprehensive integrated primary mental health care for South Africa. Pipedream or possibility? *Social science & medicine, 51*(3), 321-334.

Pollock, K. (2007). Maintaining face in the presentation of depression: constraining the therapeutic potential of the consultation. *Health:, 11*(2), 163-180.

Rahman, A., Bunn, J., Lovel, H., & Creed, F. (2007). Association between antenatal depression and low birthweight in a developing country. *Acta Psychiatrica Scandinavica, 115*(6), 481-486.

Rathod, S. D., Roberts, T., Medhin, G., Murhar, V., Samudre, S., Luitel, N. P., . . . Bhana, A. (2018). Detection and treatment initiation for depression and alcohol use disorders: facility-based cross-sectional studies in five low-income and middle-income country districts. *8*(10), e023421. doi: 10.1186/s12913-018-3716-3

Ritchie, J., Lewis, J., Nicholls, C. M., & Ormston, R. (2013). *Qualitative research practice: A guide for social science students and researchers*: Sage.

Roberts, T., Shrivastava, R., Koschorke, M., Patel, V., Shidhaye, R., & Rathod, S. D. (2019). "Is there a medicine for these tensions?" Barriers to treatment-seeking for depressive symptoms in rural India: A qualitative study. *Social science & medicine*, 112741.

Ross, L. E., Sellers, E., Gilbert Evans, S., & Romach, M. (2004). Mood changes during pregnancy and the postpartum period: development of a biopsychosocial model. *Acta Psychiatrica Scandinavica, 109*(6), 457-466.

Rost, K., Smith, R., Matthews, D. B., & Guise, B. (1994). The deliberate misdiagnosis of major depression in primary care. *Archives of family medicine, 3*(4), 333-337.

Schwenk, T. L., Klinkman, M. S., & Coyne, J. C. (1998). Depression in the family physician's office: what the psychiatrist needs to know: the Michigan Depression Project. *The Journal of clinical psychiatry, 59*, 94-100.

Seaburn, D. B., Morse, D., McDaniel, S. H., Beckman, H., Silberman, J., & Epstein, R. (2005). Physician responses to ambiguous patient symptoms. *Journal of general internal medicine, 20*(6), 525-530.

Simon, G. E., VonKorff, M., Piccinelli, M., Fullerton, C., & Ormel, J. (1999). An international study of the relation between somatic symptoms and depression. *New England journal of medicine, 341*(18), 1329-1335.

Smartt, C., Medhin, G., Alem, A., Patel, V., Dewey, M., Prince, M., & Hanlon, C. (2016). Fatigue as a manifestation of psychosocial distress in a low-income country: a population-based panel study. *Tropical Medicine & International Health, 21*(3), 365-372.

Stein, A., Pearson, R. M., Goodman, S. H., Rapa, E., Rahman, A., McCallum, M., . . . Pariante, C. M. (2014). Effects of perinatal mental disorders on the fetus and child. *The Lancet, 384*(9956), 1800-1819.

Stewart, R. C., Kauye, F., Umar, E., Vokhiwa, M., Bunn, J., Fitzgerald, M., . . . Creed, F. (2009). Validation of a Chichewa version of the self-reporting questionnaire (SRQ) as a brief screening measure for maternal depressive disorder in Malawi, Africa. *J Affect Disord, 112*(1-3), 126-134.

Thornicroft, G., Chatterji, S., Evans-Lacko, S., Gruber, M., Sampson, N., Aguilar-Gaxiola, S., . . . Borges, G. (2017). Undertreatment of people with major depressive disorder in 21 countries. The British Journal of Psychiatry, 210(2), 119-124.

Tylee, A., Freeling, P., Kerry, S., & Burns, T. (1995). How does the content of consultations affect the recognition by general practitioners of major depression in women? *Br J Gen Pract, 45*(400), 575-578.

Van Heyningen, T., Honikman, S., Tomlinson, M., Field, S., & Myer, L. (2018). Comparison of mental health screening tools for detecting antenatal depression and anxiety disorders in South African women. *PLoS One, 13*(4), e0193697.

Verhaak, P. F., & Bensing, J. M. (2007). GP mental health care in 10 European countries: patients' demands and GPs' responses. *The European journal of psychiatry, 21*(1), 7-16.

Vigo, D., Thornicroft, G., & Atun, R. (2016). Estimating the true global burden of mental illness. *The Lancet Psychiatry, 3*(2), 171-178.

Whiteford, H. A., Degenhardt, L., Rehm, J., Baxter, A. J., Ferrari, A. J., Erskine, H. E., . . . Johns, N. (2013). Global burden of disease attributable to mental and substance use disorders: findings from the Global Burden of Disease Study 2010. *The Lancet, 382*(9904), 1575-1586.

Williams, A., Sarker, M., & Ferdous, S. T. (2018). Cultural attitudes toward postpartum depression in Dhaka, Bangladesh. *Medical anthropology, 37*(3), 194-205.

Williams Jr, J. W., Mulrow, C. D., Kroenke, K., Dhanda, R., Badgett, R. G., Omori, D., & Lee, S. (1999). Case-finding for depression in primary care: a randomized trial*. *The American journal of medicine, 106*(1), 36-43.

Woody, C. A., Ferrari, A. J., Siskind, D. J., Whiteford, H. A., & Harris, M. G. (2017). A systematic review and meta-regression of the prevalence and incidence of perinatal depression. *J Affect Disord, 219*, 86-92. doi: 10.1016/j.jad.2017.05.003

Yeung, A., Chang, D., Gresham Jr, R. L., Nierenberg, A. A., & Fava, M. (2004). Illness beliefs of depressed Chinese American patients in primary care. *The Journal of Nervous and Mental Disease, 192*(4), 324-327.

Yonkers, K. A., Smith, M. V., Gotman, N., & Belanger, K. (2009). Typical somatic symptoms of pregnancy and their impact on a diagnosis of major depressive disorder. *Gen Hosp Psychiatry, 31*(4), 327-333.

Zegeye, A., Alebel, A., Gebrie, A., Tesfaye, B., Belay, Y. A., Adane, F., & Abie, W. (2018). Prevalence and determinants of antenatal depression among pregnant women in Ethiopia: a systematic review and meta-analysis. *BMC Pregnancy Childbirth, 18*(1), 462. doi: 10.1186/s12884-018-2101-x

Zimmermann, C., Del Piccolo, L., & Finset, A. (2007). Cues and concerns by patients in medical consultations: a literature review. *Psychological bulletin, 133*(3), 438.

World Health Organization (2008). mhGAP Mental Health Gap Action Programme: scaling up care for mental, neurological and substance use disorders. Geneva, WHO

World Health Organization (2010). mhGAP intervention guide for mental, neurological and substance use disorders in non-specialized health settings: mental health Gap Action Programme (mhGAP)

World Health Organization (2011). Mental Health Atlas. Geneva, WHO

World Health Organization (2016). mhGAP intervention guide for mental, neurological and substance use disorders in non-specialized health settings: mental health Gap Action Programme (mhGAP)

Appendix

Appendix 1.1: English Information sheet - pregnant women

YOU WILL BE GIVEN A COPY OF THIS INFORMATION SHEET

"Developing antenatal maternal mental health services: Identifying depression in pregnant women attending antenatal care in Sodo district health centres, Ethiopia"

We would like to invite you to participate in this research project. You should only participate if you want to; choosing not to take part will not disadvantage you in any way. Before you decide whether you want to take part, it is important for you to understand why the research is being done and what your participation will involve. Please take time to read the following information carefully and discuss it with others if you wish. Ask us if there is anything that is not clear or if you would like more information.

Aims of the research

To understand how pregnant women with depression are identified in the current primary health care service.

Who are we recruiting?

We are including pregnant women attending antenatal care at health centres in the Sodo district.

What will happen if you agree to take part?

At first we will ask you about some symptoms or difficulties that you may be experiancing. For those women who show symptoms of depression, we will collect some data from your clinical charts about your visit today. You will also be asked basic sociodemographic questions.

Some women will be invited for further evaluation on another day by the research health professional.

In addition, you will be invited to participate in a one-to-one interview. The interview will be held at your home or health centre, whichever is convenient for you. You will be asked some questions about your understanding of the difficulties that you have, wether you have communicated to this to the PHC worker and what you think will help. The interview will last up to one hour. With your agreement, we will audio-record the interview. You will be reimbursed for your transport costs and time.

Risks of being in the study

We don't expect that the discussion will cause you any difficulties. On rare occasions, people might be upset by the questions that are being asked. If you are distressed by the questions then you do not have to answer the question. If you want to withdraw from the study at any time, you will be allowed to do so without any further questioning and there will be no negative consequences for you.

Possible benefits

We hope that the information obtained will help to improve maternal mental health service in Ethiopia.

What we will do with your data

If you take part in the interview, we will make sure that the audio-recordings do not include your name or identifying information. The notes taken during the interview also will not include your name or identifying information. The audio-recordings and notes will be kept in a locked cupboard. Once the audio-recordings have been written down, and the data has been analysed, the audio-recordings will be cleared.

Nobody except the principal investigator and research advisors will know that the information belongs to you. We will keep the questionnaires in a locked cupboard.

After the end of this study, the information you tell us may be used by other researchers, but they will not be able to identify you in any way.

Main researcher:

- Dr. Fikirte Girma

You can contact me at anytime on phone number 0911 181454.

It is up to you to decide whether to take part or not. If you decide to take part you are still free to withdraw at any time and without giving a reason.

If this study has harmed you in any way you can contact the Institutional Review Board, Addis Ababa University, using the details below for further advice and information:

Institutional Review Board, School of Medicine, Addis Ababa University

Telephone number: 0115-5538734

- You may withdraw your data from the project at any time up until it is transcribed for use in the final report.
- If you do decide to take part you will be given this information sheet to keep and be asked to sign a consent form.

Appendix 1.2: Amharic Information sheet - pregnant women

ለጥናት ተሳታፊዎች የመረጃ ቅጽ (ለነፍሰጡር እናቶች)

የዚህ የመረጃ ቅጽ አንድ ኮፒ ይሰጥወታል፡፡

<u>የጥናቱ ርዕስ : የነፍሰጡር እናቶች ድብርት ህመም ላይ ያተኮረ ጥናት</u>

በዚህ ጥናት ላይ እንዲሳተፉ ተጋብዘዋል፡፡ በጥናቱ ለመሳተፍ መወሰን ያለበወት ለመሳተፍ ከፈለጉ ብቻ ነው፡፡ በጥናቱ ለመሳተፍ ፈቃደኛ ሳይሆኑ ቢቀሩ የሚከሰትብዎት ጉዳት ወይም የሚያጡት ጥቅም አይኖርም፡፡ በዚህ ጥናት ላይ ለመሳተፍ ከመወሰንዎ በፊት ጥናቱ ለምን እንደሚካሄድና የርስዎ ተሳትፎ ምን እንደሆነ መገንዘብዎ አስፈላጊ ነው፡፡ እባክዎ የሚከተለውን መረጃ በጥንቃቄ ያንብቡ፤ አስፈላጊ ሆኖ ካገኙትም ከሌሎች ሰዎች ጋር ይወያዩበት፡፡ ግልጽ ያልሆነ ነገር ካለ ወይም ተጨማሪ መረጃ የሚፈልጉ ከሆነ ይጠይቁን፡፡

የጥናቱ ዓላማ

በአሁኑ ጊዜ በሶዶ ወረዳ ጤና ጣቢያዎች የድብርት ህመም ያላቸው ነፍሰጡር እናቶች እንዴት እንደሚለዩ ላይ ጠለቅ ያለ ግንዛቤ ለማግኘት ነው፡፡

ለጥናቱ እነማን ይመረጣሉ?

በዚህ ጥናት በሶዶ ወረዳ ጤና ጣቢያዎች የቅድመ ወሊድ ክትትል የሚያደርጉ ነፍሰጡር እናቶችን የምናካትት ይሆናል፡፡

በዚህ ጥናት ላይ በመሳተፍዎ የሚጠበቅብዎት ምንድነው?

በመጀመሪያ ስለአሎት ምልክቶች ወይንም ችግሮች ጥያቄዎች እናቀርብሎታለን:: በመቀጠልም የድብርት ህመም ምልክቶች የሚያሳዩ ከሆነ ከጤና ጣቢያ ካርዶት ላይ ስለዛሬ ጉብኝቶ አንዳንድ መረጃዎችን እንሰበስባለን:: ለእርሶ አንዳንድ መሰረታዊ ጥያቄዎችን እናቀረብሎዋለን::

አንዳንድ እናቶች በሌላ ቀን በምርምሩ ጤና ባለሞያ እንዲታዩ ግብዣ ይቀርብላቸዋል::

በተጨማሪም የአንድ ለአንድ ቃለ-መጠይቅ ላይ እንዲሳተፉ ይጋበዛሉ፡፡ ቃለ-መጠይቆቹ በጤና ጣቢያ ወይም በመኖሪያ ቤትዎ ለእርስዎ አመቺ በሆነ ቦታ የሚደረጉ ይሆናል፡፡ የአለቦት የህመም ምልክቶች እንዴት እንደሚረዱዋቸው እነዚህን የህመም ምልክቶች ለጤና ጣቢያው ባለሞያ እንዳካፈሉ እና ምን ነገሮች ያሻሽሉታል ብለው እንደሚያስቡ በሚሉት ጉዳዮች ላይ ያተኩራሉ፡፡

ቃለ-መጠይቁ እስከ አንድ ሰዓት ድረስ የሚፈጅ ይሆናል፡፡ መልካም ፈቃድዎ ከሆነም ቃለ-መጠያቁን በመቅረፀ-ድምጽ የምንቀዳ ይሆናል፡፡ ለዚህ ቃለመጠይቅ የሚያወጡት የትራንስፖርት ወጭና ሰአት ማካካሻ ይከፈልዎታል::

በጥናቱ ላይ በመሳተፍዎ ሊከሰትብዎ የሚችሉ ጉዳቶች?

በዚህ ጥናት በመሳተፍዎ ወይም ውይይቱ ማንኛውም አይነት ችግር ያደርስብዎታል ብለን አናምንም፡፡ ምንአልባት በጣም አልፎ አልፎ ተሳታፊዎች በሚነሱት ጥያቄዎች ቅሬታ ሊሰማቸው ይችላል፡፡ የሚነሳው ጥያቄ እርስዎን የማይመችዎት ከሆነ ጥያቄውን አለመመለስ ወይም ለጥያቄው መልስ አለመስጠት ይችላሉ፡፡ ከጥናቱ በማንኛውም ጊዜ መውጣት ከፈለጉ ተጨማሪ ጥያቄ ሳይጠየቁ ማቋዋረጥ ይችላሉ እርሶ ላይም ምንም አይነት አሉታዊ ነገር አያስከትልም፡፡

ሊገኙ የሚችሉ ጥቅሞች

ከዚህ ጥናት የሚገኘው መረጃ በኢትዮጵያየ እናቶችን የአዕምሮ ጤና አገልግሎትን ለማሻሻል ያግዛል፡፡

የሰጡንን መረጃ ለምን ዓይነት ዓላማ እናውለዋለን?

በመቅረፀ-ድምጽ የሚቀዳ ውይይት ላይ የሚሳተፉ ከሆነ የምንጠቀምባቸው የድምጽ መቅረጫ መሳሪያዎች የእርስዎን ስም ወይም የእርስዎን ማንነት ሊያሳውቁየሚችሉ መረጃዎች እንደማያካትቱ ከወዲሁ እናረጋግጥልዎታለን፡፡ በውይይቱ ጊዜ የሚያዘው የጽሁፍ ማስታወሻም ላይ ስምዎ ወይም የእርስዎን ማንነት የተመለከቱ መረጃዎች እንደማይካተቱ እናረጋግጥልዎታለን፡ ፡ከእርስዎ ያገኘነው በድምጽም ይሁን በጽሑፍ ማስታወሻ የተያዘ መረጃ በተቆለፈ ሳጥን ውስጥ እንዲቀመጥ ይደረጋል፡፡ ከመቅረፀ-ድምጹ የተገኘው መረጃ በጽሁፍ ከሰፈረ እና መረጃው ከተተነተነ በኋላ የድምጽ መረጃው የሚደመሰስ ይሆናል፡፡

ከፕሮጀክቱ አስተባባሪዎችና ከፕሮጀክቱ የመረጃ ማኔጀሮች በስተቀር መረጃው የርስዎ መሆኑን የሚያውቅ አይኖርም፡፡ መረጃዎቹን ቁልፍ ባለው ሳጥን ውስጥ የምናስቀምጥ ይሆናል፡፡

ይህ ጥናት ከተጠናቀቀ በኋላ የሰጡን መረጃ ሌሎች ተመራማሪዎች ሊጠቀሙበት ይችላሉ፡፡ ነገር ግን በምንም መንገድ የእርስዎን ማንነት ሊያውቁ የሚችሉበት ሁኔታ አይኖርም፡፡

ዋና ተመራማሪ፡

- ዶ/ር ፍቅርተ ግርማ

የፕሮጀክቱን ዋና ተመራማሪ ማግኘት ከፈለጉ በስልክ ቁጥር 0911181454 ማግኘት ይቾላሉ፡፡

በዚህ ጥናት ለመሳተፍ ወይም ላለመሳተፍ ሙሉ በሙሉ የእርስዎ ውሳኔ ነው፡፡ ለመሳተፍ ከወሰኑ በማንኛውም ጊዜና ምንም አይነት ምክንያት መስጠት ሳያስፈልግዎ ተሳትፎዎን ማቋረጥ ይችላሉ፡፡

በዚህ ጥናት ላይ በመሳተፍዎ የሚደርስብዎት ጉዳት ካለ የአዲስ አበባ ዩኒቨርሲቲ፣ የተቋማዊ ግምገማ ቦርድን ከስር በተጠቀሰው አድራሻ ለተጨማሪ መረጃና ምክር ማግኘት ይችላሉ፡፡

የተቋማዊ ግምገማ ቦርድ፣ የህክምና ትምህርት ቤት፣ አዲስ አበባ ዩኒቨርሲቲ-

ስልክ ቁጥር፡ 0115-5538734

- የሰጡት መረጃ ለመጨረሻ ሪፖርት ተጠናቅሮ እስካልተዘጋጀ ድረስ በማንኛውም ሠዓት ከጥናቱ እንዲወጣልዎ የመጠየቅ መብ- አለዎት፡፡
- በዚህ ጥናት ላይ ለመሳተፍ ከወሰኑ ይህ የመረጃ ቅጽ እርስዎ ጋር እንዲሆን ይሰጥወታል፤ የፈቃደኝነት መጠየቂያ ቅጹንም እንዲፈርሙ ይጠየቃሉ፡፡

Appendix 1.3: English Information sheet – PHC workers

YOU WILL BE GIVEN A COPY OF THIS INFORMATION SHEET

"Developing antenatal maternal mental health services: Identifying depression in pregnant women attending antenatal care in Sodo district health centres, Ethiopia"

We would like to invite you to participate in this research project. You should only participate if you want to; choosing not to take part will not disadvantage you in any way. Before you decide whether you want to take part, it is important for you to understand why the research is being done and what your participation will involve. Please take time to read the following information carefully and discuss it with others if you wish. Ask us if there is anything that is not clear or if you would like more information.

Aims of the research

To identify potential solutions for improving mental health care for pregnant women with depression.

Who are we recruiting?

For this study we are including health care providers who work in ANC clinics of the health centres in the Sodo district.

What will happen if you agree to take part?

You will be invited to participate in a discussion group. The discussion will take place in Bui town. There will be between 5 to 8 people in the group, with a similar background to you. The group will be asked about possible approaches to solving the problems in providing care for pregnant women with moderate to severe depression. You will be invited to contribute your opinion as part of the discussion. The discussion will take between 30 – 60 minutes and it will be audio-recorded. You will be given refreshments and reimbursed for your transport costs and time.

Risks of being in the study

We don't expect that the discussion will cause you any difficulties. On rare occasions, people might be upset by the questions that are being asked. If you are distressed by the questions then you do not have to answer the question.

Possible benefits

We hope that the information obtained will help to improve PHC based care of pregnant women with moderate to severe depression in Ethiopia.

Once the overall study is completed, we will let you know what we found, either by inviting you to a meeting or giving you a leaflet.

What we will do with your data

If you take part, we will make sure that the audio-recordings do not include your name or identifying information. The notes taken also will not include your name or identifying information. The audio-recordings and notes will be kept in a locked cupboard. Once the audio-recordings have been written down, and the data have been analysed, the audio-recordings will be cleared.

Nobody except the principal investigator and research advisors will know that the information belongs to you. We will keep the data in a locked cupboard.

After the end of this study, the information you tell us may be used by other researchers, but they will not be able to identify you in any way.

Main researcher:

- Dr. Fikirte Girma

You can contact me at anytime on phone number 0911 181454.
It is up to you to decide whether to take part or not. If you decide to take part you are still free to withdraw at any time and without giving a reason.

If this study has harmed you in any way you can contact the Institutional Review Board, Addis Ababa University, using the details below for further advice and information:

Institutional Review Board, School of Medicine, Addis Ababa University

Telephone number: 0115-5538734

- You may withdraw your data from the project at any time up until it is transcribed for use in the final report.
- If you do decide to take part you will be given this information sheet to keep and be asked to sign a consent form.

Appendix 1.4: Amharic Information sheet – PHC workers

ለጥናት ተሳታፊዎች የመረጃ ቅጽ (ለጤና ባለሞያዎች)

የዚህ የመረጃ ቅጽ አንድ ኮፒ ይሰጥወታል፡፡

<u>የጥናቱ ርዕስ : የነፍሰጡር እናቶች ድብርት ህመም ላይ ያተኮረ ጥናት</u>

በዚህ ጥናት ላይ እንዲሳተፉ ተጋብዘዋል፡፡ በጥናቱ ለመሳተፍ መወሰን ያለበወት ለመሳተፍ ከፈለጉ ብቻ ነው፡፡ በጥናቱ ለመሳተፍ ፈቃደኛ ሳይሆኑ ቢቀሩ የሚከሰትብዎት ጉዳት ወይም የሚያጡት ጥቅም አይኖርም፡፡ በዚህ ጥናት ላይ ለመሳተፍ ከመወሰንዎ በፊት ጥናቱ ለምን እንደሚካሄድና የርስዎ ተሳትፎ ምን እንደሆነ መገንዘብዎ አስፈላጊ ነው፡፡ እባክዎ የሚከተለውን መረጃ በጥንቃቄ ያንብቡ፤ አስፈላጊ ሆኖ ካገኙትም ከሌሎች ሰዎች ጋር ይወያዩበት፡፡ ግልጽ ያልሆነ ነገር ካለ ወይም ተጨማሪ መረጃ የሚፈልጉ ከሆነ ይጠይቁን፡፡

የጥናቱ ዓላማ

የድብርት ህመም ያለባቸውን ነፍሰጡር እናቶች ህክምና ማሻሻያ መንገዶችን መፈለግ ነው፡፡

ለጥናቱ እነማን ይመረጣሉ?

ለዚህ ጥናት በቅድመ ወሊድ ክትትል ክፍል የሚሰሩ የጤና ባለሙያዎችን የምናካትት ይሆናል፡፡

በዚህ ጥናት ላይ በመሳተፍዎ የሚጠበቅብዎት ምንድነው?

የቡድን ውይይት ውስጥ እንዲሳተፉ የሚጋበዙ ይሆናል፡፡የቡድን ውይይቱ ቡኢ ከተማ ውስጥ እንዲካሄድ ይደረጋል፡፡እያንዳንዱ ቡድን ከ 5-8 ሰዎችን የሚይዝ ሲሆን ተሳታፊዎችም በተቻለ መጠን ተመሳሳይ እንዲሆኑ ይደረጋል፡፡ቡድኑ ከባድ የድብርት ህመም ያለባቸውን ነፍሰጡር እናቶች ህክምና ላይ የሚገጥሙ ችግሮችን እንዴት መፍታት እንደሚቻል የተለያዩ ጥያቄዎች ይጠየቃል፡፡ሀሳብዎን በውይይቱ ላይ እንዲገልጹ ይበረታታሉ፡፡ውይይቱ ከ30 ደቂቃ እስከ አንድ ሰዓት የሚወስድ ይሆናል፡፡ውይይቱ በመቅረፀ-ድምፅ የሚቀዳ ይሆናል፡፡በውይይቱ ላይ የሻይ ቡና አገልግሎት የሚኖር ሲሆን የትራንስፖርት ወጪዎንና ያጠፉትን ጊዜ ከግምት ያስገባ ገንዘብ ይሰጥዎታል፡፡

በጥናቱላይበመሳተፍዎሊከሰትብዎየሚችሉጉዳቶች

በዚህ ጥናት ላይ በመሳተፍዎ ወይም ውይይቱ ማንኛውንም አይነት ችግር ያደርስብዎታል ብለን አናምንም፡፡ምናልባት በጣም አልፎ አልፎ ተሳታፊዎች በሚነሱት ጥያቄዎች ቅሬታ ሊሰማቸው ይችላል፡፡ የሚነሳው ጥያቄ እርስዎን የማይመችዎት ከሆነ ጥያቄውን አለመመለስ ወይም ለጥያቄው መልስ አለመስጠት ይችላሉ፡፡

ሊገኙየሚችሉጥቅሞች

ከዚህ ጥናት የሚገኘው መረጃ በኢትዮጵያ የነፍሰጡር እናቶችን የድብርት ህመም ህክምና አገልግሎትን ለማሻሻል ያግዛል፡፡

አጠቃላይ ጥናቱ ከተጠናቀቀ በኃላ በጥናቱ የሚገኘውን ውጤትበስብሰባወይም በህትመቶች አማካይነት የምናሳውቅዎ ይሆናል፡፡

የሰጡንን መረጃ ለምን ዓይነት ዓላማ እናውለዋለን?

በመቅረፀ-ድምጽ የሚቀዳ ውይይት ላይ የሚሳተፉ ከሆነ የምንጠቀምባቸው የድምጽ መቅረጫ መሳሪያዎች የእርስዎን ስም ወይም የእርስዎን ማንነት ሊያሳውቁ የሚችሉ መረጃዎች እንደማያካትቱ ከወዲሁ እናረጋግጥልዎታለን፡፡ በውይይቱ ጊዜ የሚያዘው የጽሁፍ ማስታወሻም ላይ ስምዎ ወይም የእርስዎን ማንነት የተመለከቱ መረጃዎች እንደማይካተቱ እናረጋግጥልዎታለን፡፡ ከእርስዎ ያገኘነው በድምጽም ይሁን በጽሑፍ ማስታወሻ የተያዘ መረጃ በተቆለፈ ሳጥን ውስጥ እንዲቀመጥ ይደረጋል፡፡ ከመቅረፀ-ድምጹ የተገኘው መረጃ በጽሁፍ ከሰፈረ እና መረጃው ከተተነተነ በኋላ የድምጽ መረጃው የሚደመሰስ ይሆናል፡፡

ከፕሮጀክቱ አስተባባሪዎችና ከፕሮጀክቱ የመረጃ ማኔጀሮች በስተቀር መረጃው የርስዎ መሆኑን የሚያውቅ አይኖርም፡፡ መረጃዎቹን ቁልፍ ባለው ሳጥን ውስጥ የምናስቀምጥ ይሆናል፡፡

ይህ ጥናት ከተጠናቀቀ በኋላ የሰጡን መረጃ ሌሎች ተመራማሪዎች ሊጠቀሙበት ይችላሉ፡፡ ነገር ግን በምንም መንገድ የእርስዎን ማንነት ሊያውቁ የሚችሉበት ሁኔታ አይኖርም፡፡

ዋና ተመራማሪ፤

- ዶ/ር ፍቅርተ ግርማ

- የፕሮጀክቱን ዋና ተመራማሪ ማግኘት ከፈለጉ በስልክ ቁጥር 0911181454 ማግኘት ይቻላሉ፡፡

በዚህ ጥናት ለመሳተፍ ወይም ላለመሳተፍሙሉ በሙሉ የእርስዎ ውሳኔ ነው፡፡ ለመሳተፍ ከወሰኑ በማንኛውም ጊዜና ምንም አይነት ምክንያት መስጠት ሳያስፈልግዎ ተሳትፎዎን ማቋረጥ ይችላሉ፡፡

በዚህ ጥናት ላይ በመሳተፍዎ የሚደርስብዎት ጉዳት ካለ የአዲስ አበባ ዩኒቨርሲቲ፣ የተቋማዊ ግምገማ ቦርድን ከስር በተጠቀሰው አድራሻ ለተጨማሪ መረጃና ምክር ማግኘት ይችላሉ፡፡

የተቋማዊ ግምገማ ቦርድ፣ የህክምና ትምህርት ቤት፣አዲስ አበባ ዩኒቨርሲቲ

ስልክ ቁጥር፡ 0115-5538734

- የሰጡት መረጃ ለመጨረሻ ሪፖርት ተጠናቅሮ እስካልተዘጋጀ ድረስ በማንኛውም ሠዓት ከጥናቱ እንዲወጣልዎ የመጠየቅ መብት አለዎት፡፡

- በዚህ ጥናት ላይ ለመሳተፍ ከወሰኑ ይህ የመረጃ ቅጽ እርስዎ ጋር እንዲሆን ይሰጥወታል፤ የፈቃደኝነት መጠየቂያ ቅጹንም እንዲፈርሙ ይጠየቃሉ፡፡

Appendix 2.1: English Consent form - pregnant women

"Developing antenatal maternal mental health services: Identifying depression in pregnant women attending antenatal care in Sodo district health centres, Ethiopia"

Statement of Consent

I have read the participant information sheet or had it read for me. All my questions have been answered. I have read or been told about the purpose and safety of the study, what will be done and the risks and benefits of the study. I agree to be in the study.

I agree for my interview to be audio-recorded. YES NO

____________________ ________________ ______________

Name of participant Signature/ thumbprint* Date

*In case the participant is not able to read this form or sign their name, this attests that the consent form has been read and explained accurately by a member of the research staff in the presence of an independent witness, and that the participant has affixed their thumbprint as consent.

I ____________________________________agree that the research project named above has been explained to ________________________________ (participant) to his/her satisfaction and that he/she agrees to take part in the study. Both the notes written above and the Information Sheet about the project have been read to him/her, and he/she understands what the research study involves.

____________________ ________________

Signature Date

________________________ _______________ ______________

Name of research staff Signature Date

Appendix 2.2: Amharic Consent form - pregnant women

የጥናት የተሳታፊ ፈቃደኝነት መጠየቂያ ቅጽ (ለነፍሰጡ እናቶች)

<u>የጥናቱ ርዕስ : የነፍሰ ጡር እናቶች ድብርት ህመም ላይ ያተኮረ ጥናት</u>

<u>የስምምነት ማረጋገጫ</u>

የመረጃ ቅጹን አንብቢያለሁ ወይም ጥናት አድራጊው አንብቦልኛል:: ያነሳኋቸው ጥያቄዎች በሙሉ ተመልሰውልኛል:: የጥናቱን አላማ፤ ደህንነትን የተመለከቱ ጉዳዮች፤ በጥናቱ ወቅት የሚሰሩ ስራዎችን እንዲሁም ጥናቱን ተከትለው ሊፈጠሩ የሚችሉ አደጋዎችንና እንዲሁም የሚገኙ ጥቅሞችን በተመለከተ አንብቤያለሁ ወይም በጥናት አድራጊው አማካኝነት ተነቦልኛል:: በዚህ ጥናት ለመሳተፍ ተስማምቻለሁ ::

ውይይታችን በመቅረፀ ድምፅ እንዲቀዳ ተስማምቻለሁ አዎአልተስማማሁም

_____________________ _____________________ _____________________

የተሳታፊ ስም ፊርማ(የ ጣት አሻራ)* ቀን

*እንደ አጋጣሚ ሆኖ ተሳታፊው ይህንን ቅጽ ማንበብ የማይችል ወይም ስሙን ጽፎ መፈረም የማይችል ከሆነ፣ይህ በአውራ ጣት አሻራ የተፈረመው የስምምነት ማረጋገጫ የስምምነት ቅጹ ለተሳተፊው/ዋ በጥናቱ ውስጥ በሚሳተፍ ሰራተኛ በገለልተኛ ምስክር ፊት ተነቦና ተብራርቶለት እንደሆነ ያረጋግጣል::

የምስክርነት ማረጋገጫ (ማንበብ ለማይችል ተሳታፊ)

እኔ _______________ከላይ ርእሱ የተገለፀው የጥናት ፕሮጀክት አላማ ለ _______________ (ተሳታፊ) በሚፈልጉት መጠን ተገልፀላቸዋል፤ በጥናቱ ለመሳተፍ ተስማምተዋል፤ ከላይ ያለው ስለፕሮጀክቱ የሚገልፅ ማብራሪያና የመረጃ ቅጹ ተነቦላቸዋል፤ እንዲሁም ጥናቱ ምን እንደሚያካትት ተረድተዋል ::

_____________________ _____________________

ፊርማ ቀን

_____________________ _____________________ _____________________

የጥናቱ ሰራተኛ ስም ፊርማ ቀን

Appendix 2.3: English Consent form – PHC workers

"Developing antenatal maternal mental health: Identifying depression in pregnant women attending antenatal care in Sodo district health centres, Ethiopia"

Statement of Consent

I have read the participant information sheet. All my questions have been answered. I have read about the purpose and safety of the study, what will be done and the risks and benefits of the study. I agree to be in the study.

I agree for our discussion to be audio-recorded. YES NO

______________________	________________	______________
Name of participant	Signature	Date
______________________	________________	______________
Name of research staff	Signature	Date

Appendix 2.4: Amharic Consent form – PHC workers

የጥናት የተሳታፊ ፈቃደኝነት መጠየቂያ ቅጽ (ለጤና ባለሞያዎች)

<u>የጥናቱ ርዕስ : የነፍሰ ጡር እናቶች ድብርት ህመም ላይ ያተኮረ ጥናት</u>

<u>የስምምነት ማረጋገጫ</u>

የመረጃ ቅጹን አንብቢያለሁ ወይም ጥናት አድራጊው አንብቦልኛል:: ያነሳኋቸው ጥያቄዎች በሙሉ ተመልሰውልኛል:: የጥናቱን አላማ፤ ደህንነትን የተመለከቱ ጉዳዮች፤ በጥናቱ ወቅት የሚሰሩ ስራዎችን እንዲሁም ጥናቱን ተከትለው ሊፈጠሩ የሚችሉ አደጋዎችንና እንዲሁም የሚገኙ ጥቅሞችን በተመለከተ አንብቤያለሁ ወይም በጥናት አድራጊው አማካኝነት ተነቦልኛል:: በዚህ ጥናት ለመሳተፍ ተስማምቻለሁ ::

ውይይታችን በመቅረፀ ድምፅ እንዲቀዳ ተስማምቻለሁ አዎ/አልተስማማሁም

________________	________________	________________	
የተሳታፊ ስም	ፊርማ		ቀን

________________	________________	________________
የጥናቱ ሰራተኛ ስም	ፊርማ	ቀን

Appendix 3.1: English IDI participants' Socio-demographic characteristics

Date	[ ][ ]/[ ][ ]/[ ][ ][ ][ ]
Patient ID	[ ][ ][ ][ ]
Interviewer ID	[ ][ ][ ]
Name of health centre	
Do you plan to stay in this district for the next two months?	Yes
	No

Demographic Information				
101	How old are you?	[ ][ ]		AGE
102	Can you read and write?	Yes	1	LIT
		No	2	
103	What type of education did you take?	Not Educated	1	EDUTYPE
		Informal Education	2	
		Formal Education	3	
104	If the answer to question 103 is formal education, highest grade completed?	[ ][ ] grade		EDUGRAD
105	How many Children do you have?	[ ][ ]		
106	What is your marital status?	Married	1	MARISTAT
		Divorced	2	
		Separated	3	
		Widowed	4	
		Single	5	
107	Is your place of residence urban or rural?	Urban	1	RES
		Rural	2	
108	What is your occupation?	House wife	1	EMP
		Farmer	2	
		Merchant/Trader	3	
		Student	4	
		Civil servant	5	
		Daily labourer	6	
		Unemployed	7	
		Other ____________________	8	
109	Compared to others in your Kebele, how do you see your economic standing?	Lower	1	RELWEAL
		Higher	2	
		Same	3	
		Don't know	88	
		Don't want to answer	99	
110	What is the gestational age, in months?	[ ] [ ] Months		GEST
111	Is this your first pregnancy?	Yes	1	PRIMIP
		No	2	
111	Is it a high risk pregnancy?	Yes Specify:____________________ ____________________	1	HIGHRISK
		No	2	

Appendix 3.2: Amharic IDI participants' Socio-demographic characteristics

ቀን	[ ][ ]/[ ][ ]/[ ][ ][ ][ ]
የተሳታፊ መለያ ቁጥር	[ ][ ][ ][ ]
የጠያቂ መለያ ቁጥር	[ ][ ][ ]
የጤና ጣቢያ ስም	
በዚህ ወረዳ ለሚቀጥሉት ሁለት ወራት ለመቆየት ያቅዳሉ?	አዎ
	አላቅድም

በቅድሚያ ስለእርስዎ አጠቃላይ መረጃ እጠይቃለሁ፡፡ በአብዛኛው ማወቅ የምፈልገው አሁን ስላሉበት ሁኔታ ነው				
101	እድሜዎት ስንት ነው?	[ ][ ]		AGE
102	ማንበብና መጻፍ ይችላሉ?	እችላለሁ	1	LIT
		አልችልም	2	
103	ምን አይነት ትምህርት ተምረዋል?	ምንም አልተማሩም	1	EDUTYPE
		መደበኛ ያልሆነ ትምህርት	2	
		መደበኛ ትምህርት	3	
104	የጥያቄ 103 መልስ መደበኛ ትምህርት ከሆነ ስንተኛ ክፍል አጠናቅቀዋል?	[ ][ ] ክፍል		EDUGRAD
105	ስንት ልጅ አሎት?	[ ][ ]		PAR
106	የጋብቻ ሁኔታ (በአሁኑ ወቅት የትዳር ሁኔታ እንዴት ነው?)	ያገባ	1	MARISTAT
		የተፋቱ	2	
		የተለያዩ (ከባል ጋር በጥል የተለያዩ)	3	
		ባል የሞተባቸው	4	
		ያላገቡ	5	
107	**የመኖሪያ ቦታ** (የሚኖሩት ቀበሌ ከተማ ነው ወይስ ገጠር?)	ከተማ	1	RES
		ገጠር	2	
108	**ስራ** (ገቢ የሚያገኙበት ስራዎ ምንድነዉ?)	የቤት እመቤት	1	EMP
		አርሶ አደር	2	
		ነጋዴ	3	
		ተማሪ	4	
		የመንግስት ሰራተኛ	5	
		የቀን ስራ (የጉልበት ሰራተኛ)	6	
		ስራ አጥ	7	
		ሌላ___________	8	
109	በቀበሌዎ ውስጥ ካሉ ሰዎች ጋር ራስዎን ሲያወዳድሩ ያለዎት ሃብት እኩል ነው፤ ይበልጣል፤ ወይንስ ያንሳል ብለው ይገምታሉ?	ያነሰ	1	RELWEAL
		የበዛ	2	
		ተመሳሳይ	3	
		አላውቅም /አላስታውስም	88	
		መልስ መስጠት አልፈለጉም	99	
110	የስንት ወር እርጉዝ ነዎት?	[ ] [ ] ወር		GEST
111	ያሁኑ እርግዝናዎ የመጀመሪያ ነው?	አዎ	1	PRIMIP
		አይደለም	2	
112	በአሁኑ እርግዝና ላይ የተገኘ ችግር አለ?	አዎ ይግለፁ___________________ ___________________	1	HIGHRISK
		የለም	2	

Appendix 3.3: English FGD participants' Socio-demographic characteristics

Date	[ ][ ]/[ ][ ]/[ ][ ][ ][ ]
Participant ID	[ ][ ][ ][ ]
FGD Number	
Location of FGD	

Demographic Information		
101	How old are you?	[ ][ ]
102	What is your gender?	Male
		Female
103	Which health centre/hospital are you from?	Buie Hospital
		Kella H/C
		Tiya H/C
		Adele H/C
		WWW H/C
		Other Specify:________________________
104	What is your educational background?	Mid wife
		Clinical nurse (diploma)
		Clinical nurse (Bsc)
		Health officer
		Other Specify:________________________
105	Do you have experience working in ANC clinic in the past one year?	Yes
		No
106	Total duration of practice as a clinician?	[ ] years
107	Do you have training on mhGAP?	Yes
		No
106	Did you ever take on-job training on mental illness/psychiatric disorders?	Yes Specify:________________________
		No

Appendix 4.1: English Patient Health Questionnaire-9 item version (PHQ-9)

Over the last two weeks, how often have you been bothered by any of the following problems?				
1-0	Did you have little interest or pleasure in doing things?	No	0	PHIL
		Yes	1	
1-1	If yes: for how many days did you feel it?	Several days	1	
		Most of the time	2	
		Nearly every day	3	
2-0	Were you have feeling down, depressed, or hopeless?	No	0	PHFS
		Yes	1	
2-1	If yes: for how many days did you feel it?	Several days	1	
		Most of the time	2	
		Nearly every day	3	
3-0	Did you have trouble falling/staying asleep or sleeping too much?	No	0	PHIS
		Yes	1	
3-1	If yes: for how many days did you have it?	Several days	1	
		Most of the time	2	
		Nearly every day	3	
4-0	Were you feeling tired or having little energy?	No	0	PHLE
		Yes	1	
4-1	If yes: for how many days did you have it?	Several days	1	
		Most of the time	2	
		Nearly every day	3	
5-0	Did you have poor appetite or overeating?	No	0	PHLR
		Yes	1	
5-1	If yes: for how many days did you have it?	Several days	1	
		Most of the time	2	
		Nearly every day	3	
6-0	Did you feel bad about yourself – or that you are a failure or have let yourself or your family down?	No	0	PHFH
		Yes	1	
6-1	If yes: for how many days did you feel it?	Several days	1	
		Most of the time	2	
		Nearly every day	3	
7-0	Did you have trouble with concentration, such as reading the newspaper or watching television?	No	0	PHDC
		Yes	1	
7-1	If yes: for how many days did you have it?	Several days	1	
		Most of the time	2	
		Nearly every day	3	
8-0	Did you move or speak so slowly that other	No	0	PHDT

	people could have noticed? Or the opposite – being so fidgety or restless that you have been moving around a lot more than usual?	Yes	1	
8-1	If yes: for how many days did you feel it?	Several days	1	
		Most of the time	2	
		Nearly every day	3	
9-0	Did you ever have thoughts that you would be better off dead or of hurting yourself in some way?	No	0	PHWD
		Yes	1	
9-1	If yes: for how many days did you have it?	Several days	1	
		Most of the time	2	
		Nearly every day	3	
10	Total for PHQ1-PHQ9	_______		**PHQTOT**
11	*If the answer to any of the above questions is yes, ask how much it has affected her day to day activities like work, self-care or interaction with others?*	Not at all	0	**PHDR**
		Mild impairment	1	
		Moderate impairment	2	
		Severe impairment	3	

If PHQ – 9 total score is 5 or above please complete the following information

1. Participants card number:___________ Phone number____________________

2. Participant's address: Kebele________ Village ______________________________

Appendix 4.2: Amharic Patient Health Questionnaire-9 item version (PHQ-9)

ማስታወሻ:አልፎ አልፎ ብቻ (2-6 ቀናት)፣ በዛላለ ጊዜ (7-11 ቀናት)፣ ከሞላ ጎደል በየቀኑ (12-14 ቀናት) መሆኑን ይግለፁ::				**Code**
ላለፉት ሁለት ሳምንታት ከነዚህ ከምዘረዝራቸው ችግሮች ውስጥ፤ የትኞቹ ደርሰውብዎት (በየትኞቹ ተቸግረው) እንደነበር እጠይቅዎታለሁ።				
1.	የእለትተእለትተግባርዎንለማከናወን (ለመስራት) ያለዎት ተነሳሽነት ወይም ፍላጎት በጣም ቀንሶ ነበር?	አዎ	1	**PHLI**
		የለም	0	
	መልሱ አዎ ከሆነ በሁለቱ ሳምንታት ዉስጥ ለምን ያህል ጊዜ ተሰማዎት?	አልፎ አልፎ ብቻ	1	
		በዛ ላለ ጊዜ	2	
		ከሞላ ጎደል በየቀኑ	3	
2.	የመከፋት፣ የመደበት ወይም ተስፋ የመቁረጥ ስሜት ይሰማዎት ነበር?	አዎ	1	**PHFS**
		የለም	0	
	መልሱ አዎ ከሆነ በሁለቱ ሳምንታት ዉስጥ ለምን ያህል ጊዜ ተሰማዎት?	አልፎ አልፎ ብቻ	1	
		በዛ ላለ ጊዜ	2	
		ከሞላ ጎደል በየቀኑ	3	
3.1	እንቅልፍ አልወስድ ብሎዎት ወይም በደንብ መተኛት አቅትቶዎት ይቸገሩ ነበር?	አዎ	1	**PHIS**
		የለም	0	
	መልሱ አዎ ከሆነ በሁለቱ ሳምንታት ዉስጥ ለምን ያህል ጊዜ ተቸገሩ?	አልፎ አልፎ ብቻ	1	
		በዛ ላለ ጊዜ	2	
		ከሞላ ጎደል በየቀኑ	3	
3.2	እንቅልፍ በዝቶብዎት ይቸገሩ ነበር?	አዎ	1	**PHOS**
		የለም	0	
	መልሱ አዎ ከሆነ በሁለቱ ሳምንታት ዉስጥ ለምን ያህል ጊዜ ተቸገሩ?	አልፎ አልፎ ብቻ	1	
		በዛ ላለ ጊዜ	2	
		ከሞላ ጎደል በየቀኑ	3	
4.	የድካም ወይም የአቅም ማነስ ስሜት ይሰማዎት ነበር?	አዎ	1	**PHLE**
		የለም	0	
	መልሱ አዎ ከሆነ በሁለቱ ሳምንታት ዉስጥ ለምን ያህል ጊዜ ተሰማዎት?	አልፎ አልፎ ብቻ	1	
		በዛ ላለ ጊዜ	2	
		ከሞላ ጎደል በየቀኑ	3	
5.1	የምግብ ፍላጎትዎ ቀንሶ ነበር?	አዎ	1	**PHLR**
		የለም	0	
	መልሱ አዎ ከሆነ በሁለቱ ሳምንታት ዉስጥ ለምን ያህል ጊዜ ቀንሶ ነበር?	አልፎ አልፎ ብቻ	1	
		በዛ ላለ ጊዜ	2	
		ከሞላ ጎደል በየቀኑ	3	
5.2	የምግብ ፍላጎትዎ ከተለመደው በላይ ጨምሮ ነበር?	አዎ	1	**PHLA**
		የለም	0	
	መልሱ አዎ ከሆነ በሁለቱ ሳምንታት ዉስጥ ለምን ያህል ጊዜ ጨምሮ ነበር?	አልፎ አልፎ ብቻ	1	
		በዛ ላለ ጊዜ	2	
		ከሞላ ጎደል በየቀኑ	3	
6.	ራስዎን የመጥላት ወይም ዋጋ የለኝም የማለት ወይም ራሴንም ሆነ ቤተሰቤን አሳዝኛለሁ የሚል ስሜት ተሰምቶዎት ነበር?	አዎ	1	**PHFH**
		የለም	0	

	መልሱ አዎ ከሆነ በሁለቱ ሳምንታት ዉስጥ ለምን ያህል ጊዜ ተሰማዎት?	አልፎ አልፎ ብቻ	1	
		በዛ ላለ ጊዜ	2	
		ከሞላ ጎደል በየቀኑ	3	
7.	በሚሰሩት ስራ ላይ ሃሳብዎን ለመሰብሰብ/ትኩረት መስጠት አስቸግርዎት ነበር? (ለምሳሌ፣ ከሰዎች ጋር ሲጨዋወቱ ትኩረት ሰጥቶ ማዳመጥ?)	አዎ	1	**PHDC**
		የለም	0	
	መልሱ አዎ ከሆነ በሁለቱ ሳምንታት ዉስጥ ለምን ያህል ጊዜ ተቸግረው ነበር?	አልፎ አልፎ ብቻ	1	
		በዛ ላለ ጊዜ	2	
		ከሞላ ጎደል በየቀኑ	3	
8.1	ለሌሎች ሰዎች እስከሚታወቅ ድረስ በእንቅስቃሴዎ ወይም በንግግርዎ በጣም ቀስ ብለው ነበር?	አዎ	1	**PHDT**
		የለም	0	
	መልሱ አዎ ከሆነ በሁለቱ ሳምንታት ዉስጥ ለምን ያህል ጊዜ ተቸግረው ነበር?	አልፎ አልፎ ብቻ	1	
		በዛ ላለ ጊዜ	2	
		ከሞላ ጎደል በየቀኑ	3	
8.2	ለሌሎች ሰዎች እስከሚታወቅ ድረስ መረጋጋት አቅቶዎት፣ አንድ ቦታ አርፎ መቀመጥ ወይም መቆም እስከማይችሉ ሆነው ነበር?	አዎ	1	**PHDS**
		የለም	0	
	መልሱ አዎ ከሆነ በሁለቱ ሳምንታት ዉስጥ ለምን ያህል ጊዜ ተቸግረው ነበር?	አልፎ አልፎ ብቻ	1	
		በዛ ላለ ጊዜ	2	
		ከሞላ ጎደል በየቀኑ	3	
9.	ከምኖር ብሞት ይሻላል ብለው አስበው ወይም ራስዎን በሆነ መንገድ ሊጎዱ አስበው ነበር?	አዎ	1	**PHWD**
		የለም	0	
	መልሱ አዎ ከሆነ በሁለቱ ሳምንታት ዉስጥ ለምን ያህል ጊዜ ተሰምቶዎት ነበር?	አልፎ አልፎ ብቻ	1	
		በዛ ላለ ጊዜ	2	
		ከሞላ ጎደል በየቀኑ	3	
10.	የ PHQ1-PHQ9 አጠቃላይ ድምር	__________		**PHQTOT**
11.	ከተዘረዘሩት ችግሮች ለአንዳቸውም አዎ የሚል መልስ ከተሰጠ የሚከተለውን ይጠይቁ፡፡ በእነዚህ ችግሮች ምክንያት ስራዎን ለመስራት፣ የቤት ሓላፊነትዎን ለመወጣት ወይም ከሰዎች ጋር ተስማምተው ለመኖር ምን ያህል አስቸጋሪ ሆኖብዎት ነበር?	በጭራሽ አልተቸገርኩም	1	**PHDR**
		በመጠኑ ተቸግሬ ነበር	0	
		በጣም ተቸግሬ ነበር	1	
		እጅግ በጣም ተቸግሬ ነበር	2	

የ PHQ – 9 አጠቃላይ ድምር 5 እና ከዛ በላይ ከሆነ የሚቀጥሉትን ይሙሉ፡፡

1. የተሳታፊ የጤና ጣብያ ካርድ ቁጥር:____________________ ስልክ ቁጥር____________________

2. የተሳታፊ አድራሻ: ቀበሌ________ መንደር/ጎጥ ________ የአከባቢ ልዩ ስም ____________

Appendix 5.1: English In-depth interview guide

Participant No	
Date of Interview	
Interviewer Name	
Interview start time	
Interview end time	

First of all, I want to thank you for taking the time to meet with me today.

1. Tell me about you current difficulties, problems or symptoms?

Prompts

- When did it start?
- What were the symptoms?
- How much does it bother you?

2. What do you think is the cause for your problems/symptoms?

Prompts

- Is it part of your pregnancy?
- Do you think it is a response to stressful life situation?
- Do you think it is an illness?

3. Did you communicate your difficulty with the ANC care provider?

Prompts

- If you did
    - How did you communicate?
    - Did you go into the details? If not, why?
    - Were you told what it is?
    - What were you told to do about it?
    - Were you happy about it?
- If you did not
    - Why did you choose not to talk about it?

4. During your ANC visit, were you given chance to talk about those symptoms?

Prompts

- Was there time for discussion?
- Were you encouraged to talk about your symptoms?
- Were you asked about the presence of symptoms?

5. What kind of things do you think will help with these difficulties?

Prompts

- Do you think something will help?
- Do you think it will improve with time?
- Do you think talking about it and sharing it to others help?
- Do you think the health workers in the ANC clinic will help?
- Do you think medications will help?

Is there anything more you would like to add? Thank you for your time.

Appendix 5.2: Amharic In-depth interview guide

የተሳታፊ መለያ ቁጥር	[ ][ ][ ][ ]
ቀን	[ ][ ]/[ ][ ]/[ ][ ][ ][ ]
የጠያቂ ስም	
የመጠይቅ መነሻ ሰአት	
የመጠይቅ መጨረሻ ሰአት	

በመጀመሪያ ጊዜዎትን ወስደው ለቃለ መጠይቁ ስለተገኙ አመሰግናለሁ፡ ፡

1. አሁን ስላሉቦት ችግሮች ወይም ምልክቶች እስቲ ይንገሩኝ?

Prompts

- መቼ ነው የጀመርዎት?
- ምልክቶቹ ምን ምን ናቸው?
- እነዚህ ምልክቶች ምን ያህል አስቸግሮዎታል?

2. እነዚህ ችግሮች/ምልክቶች በምን ምክንያት የተከሰቱ ይመስሎታል?

Prompts

- የእርግዝናዎ አካል ይመስሎታል?
- ባሉቦት የህይወት ጫናዎች ምክንያት የመጣ ይመስሎታል?
- ህመም ይመስሎታል?

3. እነዚህን ያሎትን ችግሮች ለቅድመ ወሊድ ክትትል ባለሞያዎ ነግረዋል?

Prompts

- ከነገሩ
  - መቼ ነው ለመጀመሪያ ጊዜ የተናገሩት?
  - እንዴት ለመናገር ተነሳሱ? በራሶ ተነሳሽነት ነው ወይስ በጤና ባለሞያ ጥያቄ?
  - እንዴት ነው የገለፁት?
  - ዝረዝሩን ተናግረዋል ወይ? ካልተናገሩ ለምን?
  - ምን እንደሆነ ተነግሮዎታል?
  - ምን እንዲያደርጉ ተነገሮት/ምን አርጉ ተባሉ?
  - በመናገሮ እና በተሰጦት ምላሽ ደስተኛ ነበሩ?
- ካልነገሩ
  - ላለመናገር ለምን መረጡ?

4. በቅድመ ወሊድ ክትትሎ ጊዜ ስለ ምልክቶቹ ለመናገር እድል ተሰቶዎት ነበር?

Prompts

- ለመወያየት ጊዜ ነበረ?
- ስለችግሮት/ምልክቶት እንዲናገሩ አበረታቶታል?
- ለስምልኪዮች መኖር ተጠያቀዋል?

5. ያሉዎት ችግሮች በምን መልኩ መረዳት ይችላሉ ብለው ያስባሉ?

Prompts

- ሚረዳው ነገር አለ ብለው ያስባሉ?
- በጊዜ ሂደት ይሻሻላል ብለው ያስባሉ?
- ስለጉዳዩ ማውራትና ለሌሎች ማካፈል ይረዳኛል ብለው ያስባሉ?
- በቅድመ ወሊድ ክትትል ክፍል ያሉ የጤና ባለሞያዎች ሊረድዎት ሚችሉ ይመስሎታል?
- መድሀኒቶች ሊረዶት ሚችሉ ይመስሎታል?

ሌላ መጨመር የሚፈልጉት ሃሳብ አለ?

ጊዜዎትን ወስደው ስላነጋገሩኝ በጣም አመሰግናለሁ፡ ፡

Appendix 5.3: English Focus group discussion guide

Thank you very much for agreeing to take part in this FGD.

1. Tell me about your experience in providing mental health care for pregnant woman in ANC clinics?

Prompts

- How common is the problem?
- How easy/difficult is it to identify mental health problems in women who attend ANC clinics?
- How easy/difficult is it to diagnose mental illness in women who attend ANC clinics?
- How easy/difficult is it to manage mental illness in women who attend ANC clinics?

Now let's talk specifically about depression/common mental disorders

2. Tell me about your experience in providing care for depressed pregnant woman in ANC clinics?

Prompts

- How common is the problem?
- How easy/difficult is it to identify depression in women who attend ANC clinics?
- How easy/difficult is it to diagnose major depressive disorder/moderate to severe depression in women who attend ANC clinics?
- How easy/difficult is it to manage depression in women who attend ANC clinics?

3. What are the problems you have encountered with implementation of mhGAP/providing care for maternal depression in ANC clinics?

Prompts

- In identification
- In disclosing diagnosis
- In providing treatment and follow-up

- From patient side & illness presentation
- From your side (communication, attitude) and at a system level(training, time)

Now I'll summarize and tell you what we found from the first part, i.e. from the interviews with the pregnant women. These pregnant women were having ANC follow-up in your clinics. Not all of them had depression, some had MDD and some had emotional symptoms. Some of the important findings were

- Women don't spontaneously report emotional symptoms during consultations
- Most women are willing to disclose their symptoms if asked
- Women don't think ANC clinics are the right place to seek help for their emotional symptoms
- Care in the ANC clinics focuses mostly on physical health of the mother and wellbeing of the foetus
- Depression screening is not part of care in the ANC clinics
- These women, in addition to symptoms, have psychosocial stressor like poverty, marital problems, poor support etc...

4. How expected is this finding?

Prompts

If participants have expected the result stated

- What made you anticipate this? Why do you think the patients responded in this way?
    - How did it differ from expectations and why they think it did?

5. How do you see the findings?

Prompts

- How much, in your opinion, did the care provided at the ANC clinics address the needs of the pregnant women?

6. How can we provide a better maternal mental health service at a health centre level?

Prompts

- How can we solve the identified problems?
- What can be done to improve the service at a health centre level/on the system?
- What can be done to support health care providers?
- What can we do at a community level?

Is there anything more you would like to add?

Thank you for your time.

Appendix 6.1: Ethics approval – UCT

UNIVERSITY OF CAPE TOWN
Faculty of Health Sciences
Human Research Ethics Committee

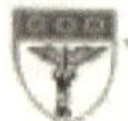

Room E52-24 Old Main Building
Groote Schuur Hospital
Observatory 7925
Telephone [021] 406 6338 · **Facsimile** [021] 406 6411
Email: nosi.tsama@uct.ac.za
Website: www.health.uct.ac.za/fhs/research/humanethics/forms

28 August 2015

HREC REF: 515/2015

Dr M Schneider
Psychiatry & Mental Health
Room 30, Building B
46 Sawkins Road, Rondebosch

Dear Dr Schneider

PROJECT TITLE: CAPE PATHWAYS FOR PREGNANT WOMEN WITH DEPRESSION WHO RECEIVE mhGAP PACKAGES OF CARE IN THE SODO DISTRICT HEALTH CENTRES, ETHIOPIA: INFORMING DEVELOPMENT OF MATERNAL MENTAL HEALTH CARE IN ANTENATAL CLINICS- (MPhil-candidate- Dr F G Bayouh)

Thank you for your letter to the Faculty of Health Sciences Human Research Ethics Committee dated 25 August 2015.

It is a pleasure to inform you that the HREC has **formally approved** the above-mentioned sub-study.

Approval is granted for one year until the 30th August 2016.

Please submit a progress form, using the standardised Annual Report Form if the study continues beyond the approval period. Please submit a Standard Closure form if the study is completed within the approval period.
(Forms can be found on our website: www.health.uct.ac.za/fhs/research/humanethics/forms)

We also acknowledge that the student, Dr FG Bayouh will be involved in this study.

Please quote the HREC REF in all your correspondence.

Please note that the ongoing ethical conduct of the study remains the responsibility of the principal investigator.

Yours sincerely

signature removed

PROFESSOR M BLOCKMAN
CHAIRPERSON, FHS HUMAN RESEARCH ETHICS COMMITTEE
Federal Wide Assurance Number: FWA00001637.
Institutional Review Board (IRB) number: IRB00001938
This serves to confirm that the University of Cape Town Human Research Ethics Committee complies to the Ethics Standards for Clinical Research with a new drug in patients, based on the Medical

HREC 515/2015

Appendix 6.2: Ethics approval - AAU

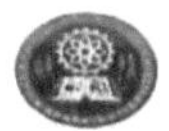

ADDIS ABABA UNIVERSITY , COLLEGE OF HEALTH SCIENCES (IRB)
አዲስ አበባ ዩኒቨርስቲ: ጤና ሳይንስ ኮሌጅ
Institutional Review Board

ANNEX 3
Form AAUMF 03-008

IRB's Decision

Meeting No: 009/15 — Date (D/M/Y): December 9, 2015
Protocol number: 048/15/Psych — Assigned No..................

Protocol Title: Care pathways for pregnant women with depression who receive mhGAP packages of care in the Sodo district health centre, Ethiopia	
Principal Investigators:	Fikirte Girma
Institute:	AAU-CHS
Elements Reviewed (AAUMF 01-008)	☑ Attached ☐ Not attached
Review of Revised Application ☐ Yes ☐ No	Date of Previous review:
Decision of the meeting:	☑ **Approved** ☐ Approved with Recommendation ☐ Resubmission ☐ Disapproved

I. Elements approved-1. Protocol Version No. ....2.............................
2. Protocol Version Date....................................
3. Informed consent Version No. ......2.....................
4. Informed Consent Version Date ....

II. Obligations of the PI-
1. Should comply with the standard international & national scientific and ethical guidelines
2. All amendments and changes made in protocol and consent form needs IRB approval
3. The PI should report SAE within 10 days of the event
4. End of the study, including manuscripts and thesis works should be reported to the IRB

III. **TO NERC** ☐

Institution Review Board (IRB) Approval: Period from 10/12/15/ to 9/12/16
Follow up report expected in
3 Months ___ 6 months ____ 9 months______ one year__√__

Chairperson, IRB
Dr. Yimtubezenash W/Amanuel
Signature
Date

www.ingramcontent.com/pod-product-compliance
Lightning Source LLC
LaVergne TN
LVHW041128150826
845673LV00007B/2233
* 9 7 8 3 3 8 4 2 3 4 1 5 5 *